THE SELF-TREATING PATIENT

Book 1

A PRACTICAL GUIDE
TO MANAGING

HEADACHE

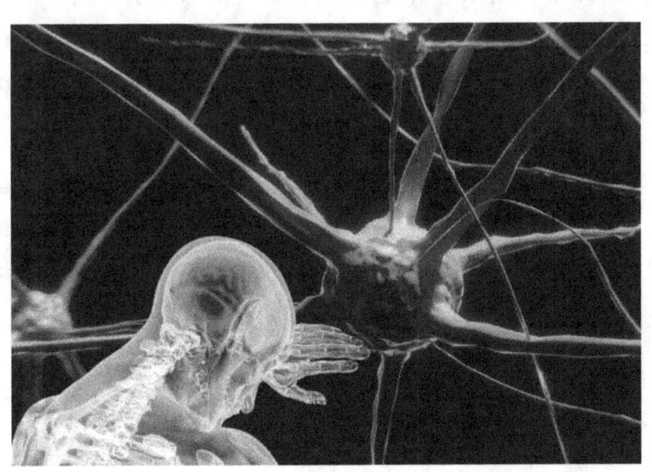

By Lovena Suson, P.T.

The Self -Treating Patient Book Series

Copyright © 2019 by Lovena Suson, P.T.

First Edition: August 2019

Graphic Design /Cover: cizcograffix@gmail.com

Dedication

This book is dedicated to Justine and Leann...

To my family, especially my siblings for unconditional love....

To friends who support and inspire...

To The TENT DOCTORS Medical Mission Team 2018

Volunteers & Sponsors

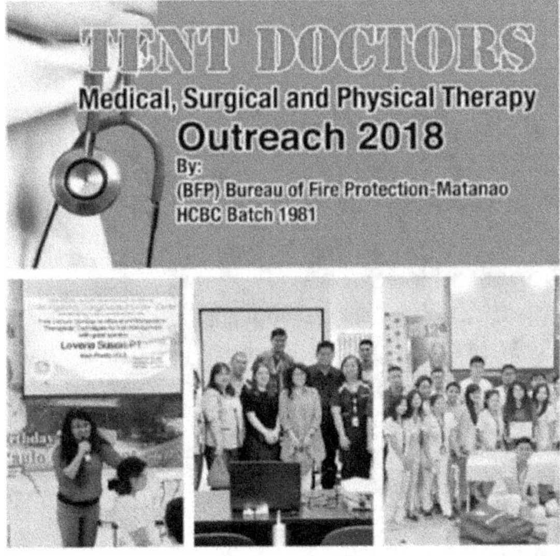

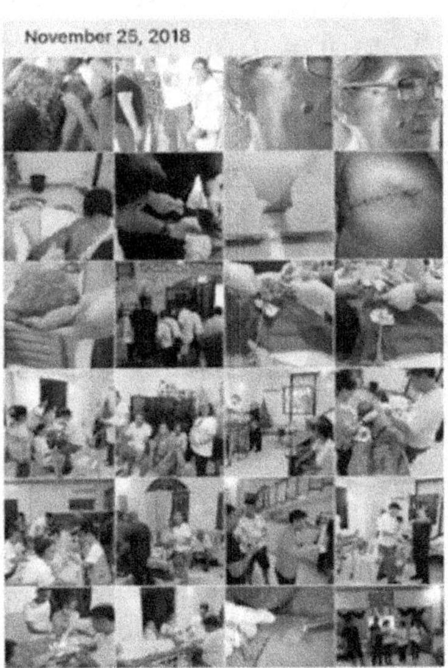

*"The best way to find yourself
is to lose yourself in the service of others".*

-Gandhi

*(A portion of the proceeds of this book will support the Author's Medical
Mission Projects)*

Regardless of gender, age, or race, we all get afflicted with headaches at some point. It is a widespread medical complaint.

Most patients referred to Physical Therapy for pain complaints *(usually of the head, neck and back)* have subsequent headaches.

This prompted sharing of relevant information to a reader who may be a headache sufferer, or who knows of one.

Many works of literature are published about headaches. Presented here are simple, helpful, practical, and unconventional approaches that are not commonly known. This will hopefully provide the sufferer with information that will aid in making informed decisions about alternative self-management.

****

FUTURE RELEASES IN THE SELF-TREATING PATIENT SERIES:

Book 1 - A Practical Guide to Managing Headache
Book 2 - A Practical Guide to Managing Pain by Improving Posture
Book 3 - A Practical Guide to Preventing Falls in the Elderly
Book 4 - A Practical Guide to Managing Menopause
Book 5 - A Practical Guide to Managing Fibromyalgia
Book 6 - A Practical Guide to Managing Parkinson's Disease
Book 7 - A Practical Guide to Managing Falls with Tai Chi
Book 8 - A Practical Guide to Managing Stress
Book 9 - The CBD Revolution: Aye or Nay?
Book 10 - Medical Marijuana: The Hype & Controversy
Book 11 - Prime Motionz - Tai Chi based Exercises for Balance
        And Fall Prevention - *developed by Lovena Suson, P.T.*

Would you like to be notified of new releases by this Author?
Get Notified Here: **https://forms.gle/kLUNQRtYsm5emZjP7**

To receive notifications for Free & Helpful E-books & Articles from this Author:
 Get Notified Here: **https://forms.gle/PzPqME3MXnKspxVi6**

Contents

Chapter 1

What Are Headaches?

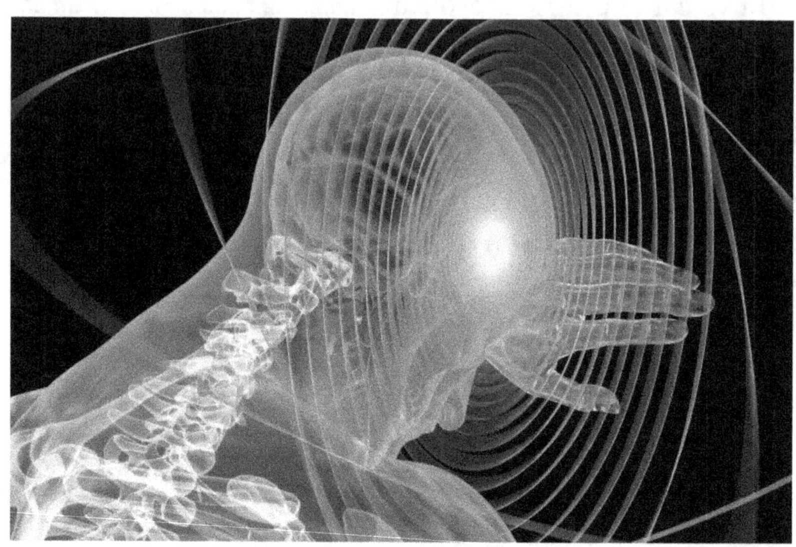

Headache is a pain that arises from the head or upper cervical region. It generates from structures that include the skull or the cerebrum. The brain itself has no nerves that perceive the sensation of pain. Bones are covered with a thin layer of tissue (periosteum), while muscles surround the skull, sinuses, eyes, and ears. Meninges arteries, veins, and nerves can get inflamed and cause a headache. The pain could be a dull ache, sharp, throbbing, constant, intermittent, mild, or intense.

Headache or head pain can be hard to detect. Primary symptoms are squeezing steady, constant, unrelenting, or intermittent pain.

The area involved can be in one section of the face or skull or can include the entire head. The typical region for pain in the body is the head.

Anatomy of Headache: How It Happens and Why?

A headache is an indicator of physical stress and emotional distress. It is also the result of specific medical disorders, including migraine, anxiety, depression, and even high blood pressure.

There exist more severe causes of headaches, such as tumors and strokes. Both are relatively rare and are not primary indicators. Discussed herein are the origins of the more classic headache types regularly experienced by sufferers.

Headache can directly cause other problems as well. It can be disabling. Statistics show that it is a common factor in work productivity. Sufferers commonly miss workdays and decrease work performance during work hours. Headaches are the third leading cause of missed school days.

People who suffer from a chronic migraine headache are unable to participate regularly with tasks of daily living. Whether from school or work, missed days and absence is prevalent. Depression can also result due to the isolation and inability to participate in social activities.

One may feel that pain comes from inside the head. However, there are no specific structures within the brain that generate pain sensation itself. It is the sensory feedback from other sources in the body transmitted to the brain.

The following will briefly explain why this symptom happens.

1. The Arteries in the Brain

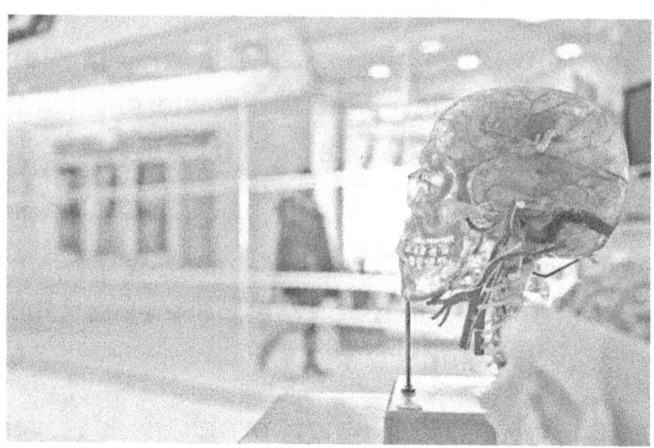

There are studies conducted on the arteries of the brain, and its role in headaches. The exact mechanism that ends in migraines is still not fully understood. There is one thing sure, however: when migraines do occur, there is dilation of the arteries. This dilation can cause inflammation of the arterial nerves.

The transmission of impulses from the nerve endings to the trigeminal ganglion causes the headache sensation.

Most pharmaceutical drugs for treating migraine symptoms are focused on the reduction of this swelling of arteries.

2. The Nerve Roots: C1, C2, C3

C1, C2, and C3 are the term for the cervical (neck) bones that these nerve roots exit from.

Often, headaches begin instantly after a head and neck injury. Whiplash or concussion can result in the uppermost nerves in the neck to become irritated. The resulting pain is on the back and top of the head. If ignored, this can lead to ongoing nerve disturbances or occipital neuralgia.

Nerves from the Upper Cervical Region

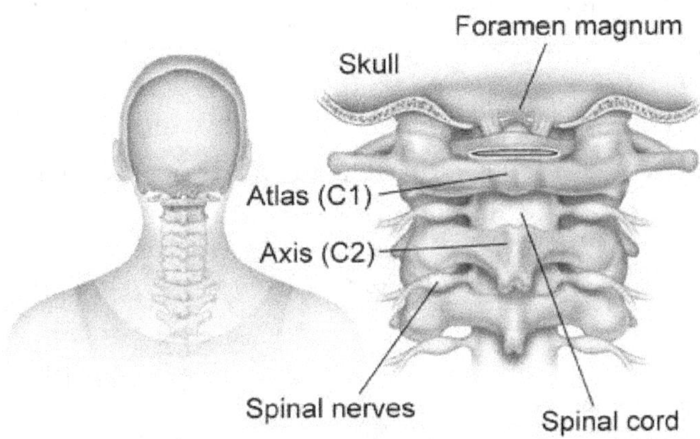

3. The Role of Meninges

The brain and spinal cord are vital organs of the central nervous system. Covering these structures are three layers of connective tissue called the Meninges. It's far probably that you recognize the term "Meningitis," which means "irritation or inflammation of the Meninges." A genuinely severe headache can be a secondary symptom of meningitis. Even when there is no meningeal infection, meninges can still contribute to headache pain.

Numerous researches has shown the connection among the sub-occipital muscles connect into the meninges. Tension on this sheath around the CNS (Central nervous system) can contribute to complications and inevitable headaches. Those dural bridges are associated with the etiology of cervicogenic problems and pain syndromes."

4. Head and Neck Muscles

A strong correlation exists in tension (type) headaches and the musculature of the neck and head. Over the years, the influence of these muscles exaggerates the problem. Specific muscles play a role in pain felt "in the head." Pain referred to the head can originate from muscles like the splenius capitis.

Patients suffering from TMJ often have correlated headaches, as well. Pain generates from the contraction of the muscles of the jaw (temporalis, master, and pterygoids)

Muscles and Structures Associated with Headaches

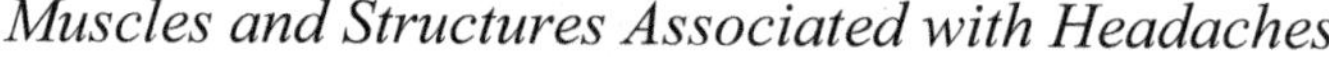

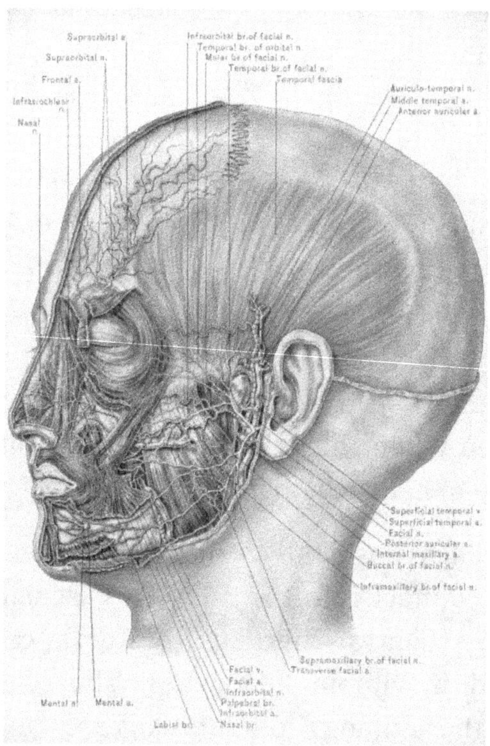

5. Dysfunction of Joints of the Neck

The joints of the neck and spine continually receive feedback from the brain. It is an integral component of posture and its role in the neurological functions of the spinal cord. Irritation results when these joints shift out of position for a more extended period (Chronic). This neck dysfunction results in "Cervicogenic" headaches. Although more difficult to classify, they are present in individuals who have had whiplash and head injuries (TBI and concussion).

6. Neurology and the Trigeminal Nerve Complex

For most head and neck pain signals, this specific bundle of nerves is the central "clearinghouse." All of the neural information from the first three spinal nerves, i.e., C1-C3, the jaw muscles, skin of the meninges, and the face is transmitted through and processed by the trigeminal complex. Trigeminal Neuralgia is a more severe form of problems that result from disturbances in this complex.

What does this mean? We can (positively) affect a person's headache disorder if we can change the function of the trigeminal complex.

Chapter 2

Causes of Headache

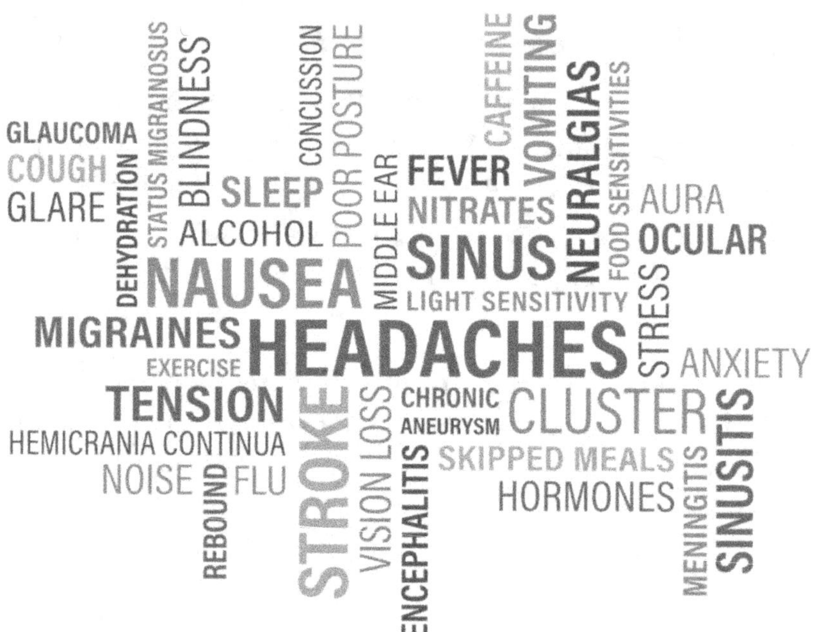

There are different factors and reasons that can bring on headaches, most of which are common in everyday life. However, problems may also be associated with severe illnesses and infections.

GENERAL CAUSES *(Not Limited to the Following)*

- Anxiety and Stress
- Dehydration
- Prolonged exposure to a computer screen, TV, or phone
- Loud Music
- Cigarette Smoking

- Alcohol Consumption
- Coffee Intake
- Irregular Meal Schedule
- Sleep Deprivation, and changes in sleep patterns
- Head Injury or Concussion
- Distance Travels or Road trips
- Hormonal changes in Teens
- Side Effects of Medications
- Vision problem

INFECTIONS THAT MAY ALSO CAUSE HEADACHES

- Flu
- Sinus infection
- Strep Throat
- Urinary Tract Infection
- Ear Infection
- Lyme Disease
- Meningitis

Chapter 3
Classification and Types of Headaches

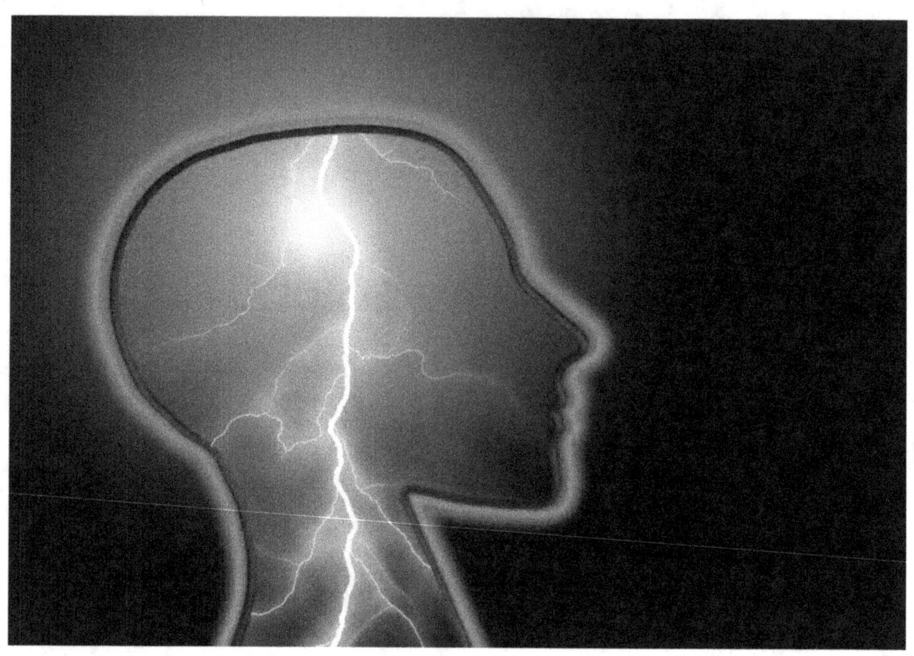

Headache pain can occur in any area of the head. This may be bilateral or occurs on only one side. There are many headache classifications:

The International Headache Society (IHS), classifies headache as PRIMARY when there are no other underlying conditions.

It is classified as SECONDARY when there is no existence of any other underlying cause.

PRIMARY HEADACHES

Primary headaches are solitary sickness or illnesses caused legitimately by the overactivity of, or problems with, structures in the head that are pain-sensitive.

These pain-sensitive structures in the Head:

- Extracranial pain-sensitive structures:
- Sinuses
- Eyes/orbits
- Ears
- Teeth
- TMJ (Temporomandibular Joint)
- Blood vessels
- 5,7,9,10 cranial nerves carry pain from this structure.

Intra-cranial pain-sensitive structures:

- Arteries of the circle of Willis and proximal rural arteries,
- Dural Venous sinuses, veins.
- Meninges.
- Dura.

This type of headaches may also result from changes in chemical activity in the brain. Frequent primary headaches include migraines, cluster headaches, and tension headaches.

SECONDARY HEADACHES

Secondary headaches are signs and symptoms that show up when another condition stimulates the pain-sensitive nerves of the head. In different words, headache signs attribute to some other reason. Usually, secondary headaches are the signs and symptoms of an injury or an underlying illness. For instance, due to increased pressure or infection in the sinuses, sinus headaches are considered a secondary problem.

Many factors can be the reason for secondary headaches; some of which are the following:

- Hangovers from Drinking Alcohol
- Tumors in the Brain
- Blood Clots
- Intracranial Bleeding
- "Brain freeze," or ice-cream headaches
- Poisoning by Carbon Monoxide
- Concussions
- Dehydration
- Glaucoma
- Bruxism (Teeth - grinding at night)
- Flu Virus
- Abuse of Pain Medications
- Anxiety and Panic attacks
- TIA/CVAs and other cerebrovascular disorders

Because headaches can indicate other conditions, it is critical to seek medical attention.

If disregarded, they become progressively severe, constant, and persistent.

When you experience intense pain, significant than past migraines, fail to improve with medication, or accompanied by other symptoms (such as perplexity, fever, sensory changes, and firmness in the neck), then seek medical attention immediately.

****

CLASSIFICATION OF HEADACHES

The International Headache Society in 2013 released its most recent grouping or classification framework for headaches.

A significant number of individuals suffer from headaches, and treatment can be very challenging.

The Headache Society theorized that the new classification would enable health care professionals to diagnose headache type and provide better alternatives for treatment accurately.

The rules are broad, and the Headache Society suggests that Health care professionals usually consult the regulations for diagnosis.

There are three classifications of headaches based on pain source:

- Primary Headaches
- Secondary Headaches
- Cranial Neuralgias, Facial Pain, and Other Headaches

A patient, however, can also exhibit consistent signs and symptoms with two or more types of headaches simultaneously.

Primary Headaches and its Types:

Primary headaches are those that have no structural or metabolic abnormality.

- Migraine
- Tension-type Headache
- Cluster Headaches
- Trigeminal Autonomic Cephalgias
- A variety of other less frequent problems.

Primary headaches can affect the quality of life. A few people have intermittent problems that resolve quicker than others. Headaches are usually non-threatening. However, they can demonstrate symptoms that mimic a cerebrovascular incident.

MIGRAINE HEADACHE

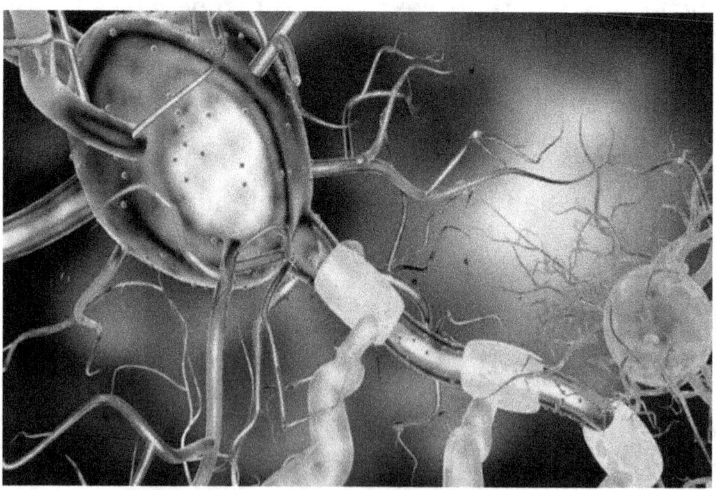

A migraine is extreme pulsing from inside the head. This pain can persist for quite a long time and restrict everyday activities. The indications and symptoms of migraine include throbbing, which usually begins on one side of the head. Sensitivity to light and noise, nausea, and emesis are usual reactions to migraines.

Specific compounds and situations are responsible for triggering and initiating a migraine. They mostly occur more in women, i.e., 75% approximately, and can affect the person's ability to perform daily activities.

SYMPTOMS OF MIGRAINE:

Symptoms of migraines include unilateral throbbing pain on one side of the head.

The pain can radiate to the eyes, forehead, or temple, resulting in nausea, vomiting, visual disturbances like diplopia, and sensitivity to ordinary light or mild exertion.

Epidemiology:

- Migraine affects 10-15% of the general population, Females > Males
- Migraine is responsible for 10-20% of all headaches in adults.
- Its mean frequency is 1.2/month.
- Its mean duration is 24 hours (untreated).
- 10% is always with aura, >30% is sometimes with aura.
- The usual age onset is about 15-35 years.

Family History:

70% of patients are likely to have family members or relatives with the same problems.

Migraine with Aura:

"Classical" headaches start with an aura. As an example: seeing visual field changes (dots, wavy lines, blurriness) about an hour or less before the onset of pain begins. This type afflicts twenty (20%) of individuals.

Classical auras do not happen in all patients.

*25% of migraine patients can experience the prodromal stage.

* The prodromal stage happens about 24 hours prior pain build-up.

*The prodromal stage comprises of mood changes (depressed, hyperactivity, irritability) and sensation of odd scents or tastes. Others also feel worn out, tired, and tense.

Migraine Triggers:

*Stress and anxiety

*Emotions

*Lack of food and sleep

*Flashing light

*Hormonal changes

*Tyramine produced from the amino acid tyrosine

*Alcohol and caffeine

Individuals who take alcohol and caffeine regularly are prone to develop a headache when they quit intake or decrease the frequency of consumption.

Diagnosing Migraine:

The clinical history and symptoms are usually adequate to diagnose migraines. Most practitioners will conduct a CT (Computed Tomography), or MRI (Magnetic Resonance Imaging) brain scan to determine other causes (brain tumor or intracranial hemorrhage).

Treatments and Medications for Migraine

*Over the counter medicines (OTC) like aspirin, naproxen sodium, ibuprofen, and acetaminophen, etc. (It is not advisable to overuse these)

*Triptans (Amerge, Axert, Frova, Imitrex, Maxalt, Relpax, Treximet, and Zomig)

*Analgesics (aspirin 900mg, ibuprofen 400mg, paracetamol 1000mg, etc.)

*Ergotamines (Cafergot, Migergot, or Migrana)

Alternative Therapies:

Biofeedback: Biofeedback is a technique used to prevent migraines by reducing migraine triggers like stress and early symptoms like muscle tension.

Acupuncture: Acupuncture, the Chinese method of treating illnesses by inserting needles into a specific body part to reduce or stop the pain.

Patients respond well to this method, although studies on acupuncture are still not definite and clear. Some physicians do not recommend this treatment because the results are so variable.

But because it benefits some patients, it is another treatment to consider.

****

TENSION TYPE HEADACHES

The most common primary headache is tension headaches. This type affects women more than adult males.

According to the World Health Organization, daily tension headaches afflict one in twenty individuals in the world.

This pain may range from mild to moderate, and such an occurrence can come and go unpredictably.

What Causes Tension Headaches?

The most frequently occurring type of headache is tension headaches. Their cause isn't entirely known. Likely reasons are hypertonicity of the muscles that cover the skull. The tissues covering the scalp can become inflamed and go into spasm.

The structures which pain can originate from are the occipital and nuchal region where the upper trapezius inserts the muscles at the temples which move the jaw and the forehead.

The definitive cause of tension headaches is difficult to determine. There is little research done to confirm the cause. Some believe that physical stress on the muscles of the head is a cause of tension headaches. These stressors cause masticatory muscles to go into spasm and teeth clenching.

Other physical stressors include strenuous and prolonged manual labor, sitting at a desk, concentrating on a computer for long.

Tension headaches can also result from emotional stresses and can lead to tension, hypertonicity in the head and neck musculature.

Signs and Symptoms of Tension Headaches

Pain starting from the back of the head and upper neck and frequently manifests as a band-like tightness or pressure. It can also spread to encircle the entire head.

Severe pressure is felt at the temples and above the eyebrows where the temporalis and frontal muscles are.

The pain is bilateral, affecting both sides of the head. The intensity may vary. Usually, it is not disabling, and the sufferer can still easily continue with daily activities.

The pain is not associated with an aura, nausea, vomiting, or sensitivity to light and sound.

The pain can occur intermittently with no specific and predictable pattern.

But with some individuals, this can occur **frequently** and even **daily.**

Despite the headache, this pain allows people to function as usual. However, quality of work or performance declines. Students cannot focus, have decreased attention span, and poor concentration. Restlessness can happen and is very common.

Diagnosing Tension Headaches:

The history provided by the patient is key to diagnosing any headache. Questions are asked frequently by health care professionals before diagnosis. Those questions will define the quality, quantity, and duration of the pain, as well as any associated symptoms.

With tension headaches, there is mild-to-moderate pain experienced by the patient on both sides of the head. People with tension headaches describe an ache that is not throbbing, nor is it worsened with tasks or chores. There are usually no associated symptoms like nausea, vomiting, or light sensitivity.

Physical and neurological examinations are both crucial for diagnosis. There is also tenderness in the muscles of the neck and scalp. If a healthcare professional detects an abnormality upon neurologic exam, the determination of tension headache is on hold until the potential for other causes is ruled out.

TREATMENT:

Treatment of Tension Headaches include the following:

*OTC (over-the-counter) pain medications are mostly used to control tension headaches.

*These medications also worked well for some people:

*Aspirin

*Ibuprofen (Motrin, Advil)

*Acetaminophen (Tylenol, Panadol)

*Naproxen (Aleve)

Other supportive treatments are also available if these medications fail:

*Physical therapy

*Massage Therapy

*Chiropractic Care

*Biofeedback (Also known as progressive relaxation where instruments are used to monitor a patient's response as shown in muscle tension or temperature in the skin)

*Stress management.

****

CLUSTER HEADACHES

The most severe form of headaches is cluster headaches as they tend to happen in groups, thus the term cluster headaches. During a cluster period, one may experience them one to three times each day. This can last two weeks to 3 months. Every attack of cluster headache lasts for about 15 minutes to 3 hours. They can wake the patient up in the middle of the night.

A sufferer may be in remission for a long time, even years, only to recur later. Men are three to multiple times bound to get them as compared to ladies.

In cluster headaches, you could have intense burning or piercing pain behind or around one eye. It can also surface as a throbbing or constant pain. People with cluster headaches cannot sit still, but will often pace during an attack. The pain is so intense and severe enough to cause distress, ptosis, redness, and teary eyes.

The nostril on the same side gets congested or runny as well.

What Causes Cluster Headaches?

The reason for Cluster headaches is dubious. It might be because of the arrival of the chemical compounds, histamine, and serotonin in the brain. A region located at the base of the brain called the hypothalamus might be a source.

Despite its small size, the hypothalamus has many functions. One of which is body temperature regulation. It maintains balance in the body's physiological cycles. When there is a disruption in these cycles, cluster headaches can be triggered.

As observed in the brain of cluster headache sufferers (during an active attack), abnormalities were present in the brain scan.

MORE FACTS ABOUT CLUSTER HEADACHES

1. t's believed to be hereditary
2. Changes in sleep patterns can be a trigger
3. Can be caused by certain medications like Nitroglycerine (prescribed for heart disease)
4. Cigarette smoking, alcohol, and some foods like chocolate, and processed foods (like smoked meats) also potentially cause these headaches.

WHEN CLUSTER HEADACHES ATTACK:

1. Pain typically occurs once or twice daily during the period when the cluster headache occurs. A few patients may experience pain more than twice every day.
2. Each episode of a cluster headache lasts anywhere from 30 to 60 minutes.
3. Attacks, in general, will happen at a similar time each day, and often wake the patient up from sleep at night.
4. The pain experienced is located around or behind one eye. This is typically excruciating and often described by patients as a hot poker.

5. The affected eye becomes red, inflamed, and watery. The nose also gets congested and runny on the affected side.

HOW ARE CLUSTER HEADACHES DIAGNOSED?

Diagnosing cluster headaches is made by taking a patient history. The description of pain and its clock-like recurrence is usually sufficient to make the findings.

Once diagnosed, one usually finds the patient in a pain crisis — the eyes and nose water when examined amid an attack. If the physical examination is routine, the diagnosis will be contingent upon history whether the patient has received care in the past or not.

CLUSTER HEADACHE TREATMENTS

Treatment of cluster headache takes trial and error to find the specific treatment regimen that will work for each patient.

It is because they are often difficult to treat. When symptom recurs daily, two treatments are needed. The first is to control and prevent the first episode, and the second prevents the ensuing headache.

Initial treatment of cluster headaches includes one or more of the following options:

1. *Inhalation of high concentrations of oxygen (not useful for chronic problems)
2. *Injection of triptan medications namely Triptan (Imitrex), Zolmitriptan (Zomig), and Rizatriptan (Maxalt)
3. *Spraying or dripping lidocaine, a local anesthetic into a patient's nostrils
4. *Dihydroergotamine (DHE, Migranal), (a medication that causes vasoconstriction)
5. *Caffeine.

6. *Triptan Drugs
7. *Oxygen Therapy
8. *Vagus Nerve Stimulation/Non-invasive

PREVENTION AND TREATMENT OF HEADACHE AND PAIN THAT FOLLOW:

*Calcium channel blockers, like verapamil (Calan, Verelan, Verelan PM, Isoptin, Covera-HS) and diltiazem (Cardizem, Dilacor, Tiazac);

*Prednisone (Deltasone, Liquid Pred);

*Antidepressant Medications;

*Lithium (Eskalith, Lithobid);

*Antiseizure drugs (Valproic acid, Divalproex (Depakote, Depakote ER, Depakene, Depacon), and Topiramate (Topamax).

CAN CLUSTER HEADACHES BE PREVENTED?

Cluster headache episodes may be spaced years apart. This makes the first episode challenging to determine. For this reason, daily medication is not necessary.

Lifestyle changes reduce the risk of a cluster headache flare-up.

Future episodes of cluster headache can also be prevented by stopping smoking and decreasing the intake of alcohol.

****

WHAT ABOUT SECONDARY HEADACHES?

Secondary headaches have structural and metabolic abnormalities.

*Extracranial (Factors outside of the head)

*Intracranial (factors within the skull)

*Metabolic disorders

WHAT CAUSES SECONDARY HEADACHES?

Headache is a symptom associated with many illnesses. The headache itself can be the primary issue.

Secondary headaches, however, can be attributed to an underlying disease or injury.

Symptom control is essential in conjunction with efficient diagnostics to identify the underlying condition. Some causes of a secondary headache may be potentially life-threatening and fatal.

Early diagnosis and treatment are imperative, so irreversible damage can be avoided.

The International Headache Society lists eight categories of secondary headache. These are:

1. Head and Neck Trauma.
2. Vascular (diseases in the head and neck)
3. Non-vascular problems in the brain
4. Medications and drugs, including withdrawal from those drugs.
5. Infections
6. Changes in the Body Environment

7. Problems with the eyes, ears, nose, throat, teeth, sinuses, and neck.

HOW TO DIAGNOSE SECONDARY HEADACHES

Diagnosis of Secondary headaches begins appropriately with a thorough history taking. Physical Examination, laboratory workup, and radiologic tests are also completed as appropriate.

In some cases, a health care professional may decide to treat a specific cause without waiting for tests to confirm the diagnosis.

This scenario is when the patient is unconscious, in critical condition, and has unstable, and unstable vital signs.

As an example: a patient with headache, fever, stiff neck and confusion may have meningitis. Meningitis can be rapidly fatal. Antibiotic therapy is initiated before blood tests, and a lumbar puncture is performed to confirm the diagnosis.

Another example is when the presence of a brain tumor or subarachnoid disease is suspected.

However, the benefit of early antibiotics outweighs the risk of not being provided promptly.

TESTING FOR SECONDARY HEADACHES

Patient history and physical examination can determine the cause of secondary headaches. It is crucial for patients who experience severe symptoms to seek medical care and allow for assessment and appropriate treatment of their condition.

Tests conducted for the diagnosis of underlying disease will depend upon the doctor's evaluation. The process will also determine specific conditions as the cause (secondary diagnosis).

Standard tests conducted include the following:

1. Blood Tests
2. Computerized Tomography (CT scan) of the neck
3. Magnetic Resonance Imaging (MRI) scans of the head.
4. Lumbar Puncture (spinal tap)

Chapter 4

Common Treatments for Headache

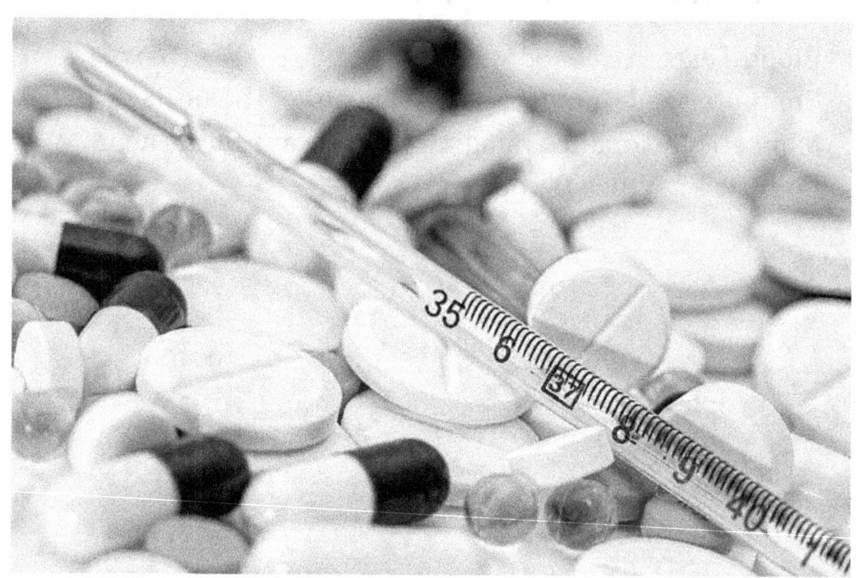

The Most Common Interventions for Treating Headaches:

1. Rest and pain relief medications.
2. Seeking medical help.
3. Electronic medical devices are now used to treat severe headaches.
4. Counseling.
5. Stress Management.
6. Biofeedback.
7. Botox – is a neurotoxin poison from bacteria Clostridium Botulinums. Indicated for migraine and tension type headaches involve injections of thirty to forty shots equally on each side of the head;Usually, about one time every twelve weeks or so. I

will not get into details about this treatment. Do consult your physician if this is an appropriate treatment for you.

Your doctor can formulate a treatment plan to meet your specific needs according to the type and frequency of your headache.

WHEN TRADITIONAL TREATMENT DOESN'T HELP

Alternative Treatments always get clearance and approval from your physician before embarking on alternative treatments. Make sure you have received the proper medical care from a physician.

KNOWN AND CONVENTIONAL ALTERNATIVE APPROACHES

1. Acupuncture
2. Cognitive Behavior Therapy (CBT) by a Mental Health Counselor
3. Herbal and Nutritional Health Products
4. Hypnosis
5. Meditation

Research has not provided evidence to confirm that all these methods work. Sometimes, a headache may result from a deficiency of a particular nutrient or nutrients.

Magnesium and specific B vitamins are one of the few.

Nutrition deficiencies, such as poor-quality diet, underlying malabsorption issues, or other medical conditions, should also be addressed for prevention.

ARE THERE HOME REMEDIES FOR HEADACHES?

HOME REMEDIES

(When conventional treatment is not enough)

Steps can be taken to reduce the risk of headaches, and ease symptoms if they do occur:

1. Application of a heating pad or ice pack to the head and neck.
2. Avoiding extreme temperatures for the risk of burns.
3. Avoiding stressors, where possible, and develop healthy coping strategies for unavoidable stress.
4. Eating regular meals, taking care to maintain stable blood sugar.
5. A hot shower can help. A hot shower finished with a cold shower was also believed to improve the body into balance. In some instances, however, hot water exposure may trigger headaches.
6. Exercising regularly and getting enough rest.
7. Regular and restful sleep facilitates stress reduction and improve health and well-being.
8. Most patients with migraine headaches get relief after resting in a dark room and falling asleep.

Prescription medications are available to treat the symptoms. Some remedies are to treat symptoms of nausea and vomiting.

Those with migraine headaches often have a system of self-treatment at home. I have learned a lot from my patients who shared how they manage headaches on their own.

PRACTICAL STRATEGIES TO MANAGING HEADACHES

1. First and foremost, treating a headache with medication as prescribed by a physician or specialist.
2. Behavioral Treatment or Therapy
3. Massage
4. Relaxation Training
5. Lying down in a dark and quiet room
6. Hot or cold compresses on the head and neck
7. Meditations
8. Cognitive-behavioral therapy (CBT)
9. WATER, WATER, AND MORE WATER! Getting the ideal dose of 8 glasses a day helps!

****

Chapter 5

After Seeing My Doctor, What Else Can I Do?

This is the chasm where a patient is left once conventional treatment options have been explored. There is still that black hole where a patient is left to deal with the headache symptoms that come and go. This is where a patient becomes - THE SELF TREATING PATIENT.

After all, one still has to deal with the chores and tasks of daily living. Headache or not, meals have to be prepared, pets and children need to be taken care of, and job tasks have to be done. Even a "minor" headache can take the joy out of enjoying quality time with family and social activities.

"Some pain you can distance yourself from; but a headache sits right where you live."

-Mark Lawrence

A HEADACHE DIMINISHES QUALITY OF LIFE

I know. I get it. I see it all the time.

That vice on your head keeps tightening by the minute, and one still has to do what needs to be done. Suddenly, the most menial of tasks become arduous.

I admire the resilience of headache sufferers I have had the privilege of working with. They stayed positive. Some have shared unconventional strategies, home remedies, tricks, and options that I will share in this book.

The information shared in this section is meant to serve as a GUIDE. So, one may be able to explore options and make informed decisions on how to manage symptoms. Some mentioned here may not be appropriate or help specific individuals. But if a few will find this information useful in managing headaches, my purpose for this book has been realized. For that, I am hopeful.

I endeavored to keep details simple, as there are a plethora of resources available to further learn and study options.

****

RELEVANCE OF POSTURAL CORRECTION IN HEADACHES

One would notice that this is number one on my list.

I have blogged about bad posture, *"weighing us down."*

(You may refer to Book 2 of my series:

The Self-Treating Patient, A Practical Guide To Managing Pain By Improving Posture)

This cannot be any farther from the truth.

I am adamant and truly emphatic about this to patients, even after you have seen the most skilled clinical practitioners. If posture is not corrected, the care provided at the clinic will be fruitless.

Ninety percent of patients we see at the clinic have lousy posture. They come in for back, neck, shoulder, and even leg pains. Bad posture begets pain.

As I have written in one of my Blogs:

"Biomechanically speaking, for every inch of forwarding deviation of the head, there is an equivalent additional load of about 15 to 30 pounds placed on these muscles.

This doubles the weight of the head, forcing these muscles to contract for prolonged periods throughout the day. Muscles can only contract for a specific period before fatigue sets in."

Muscle spasms are then caused by this muscle overuse and fatigue. Dehydration and abnormalities in the body's electrolyte levels are also known causes of muscle spasms.

The simplest motion of aligning your head and neck back towards your mid-line eliminates this excessive load and induces the relaxation of the muscles of the head and neck.

When muscles of the head, neck, shoulders and upper back are relaxed, pressure to the head decreases. Proper posture can aid in the prevention of headaches.

IDEAL POSTURE FOR RELAXATION AND PAIN PREVENTION

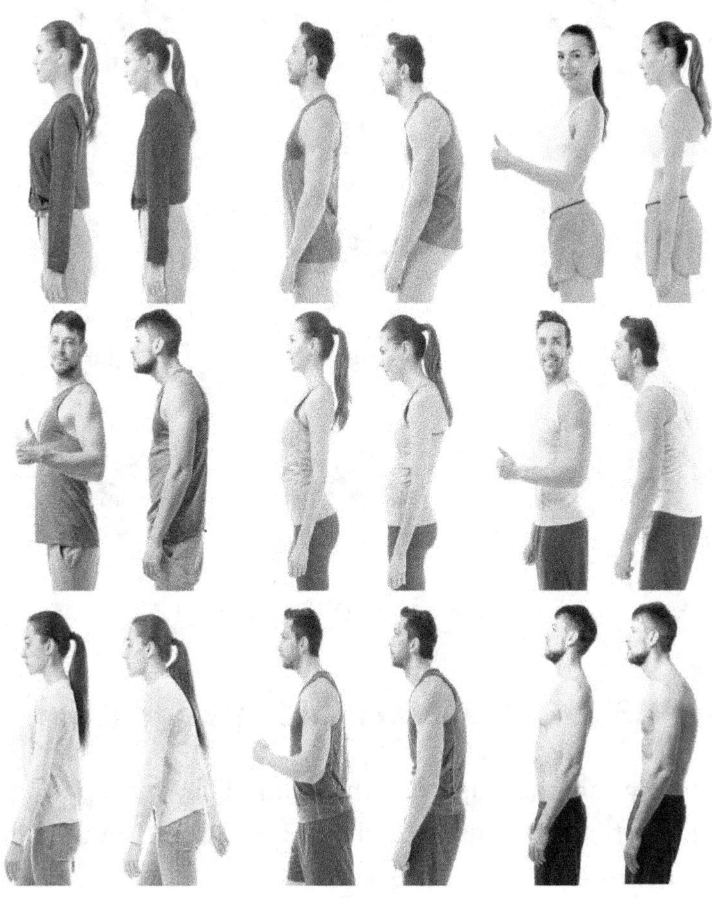

Posture during Standing and Walking

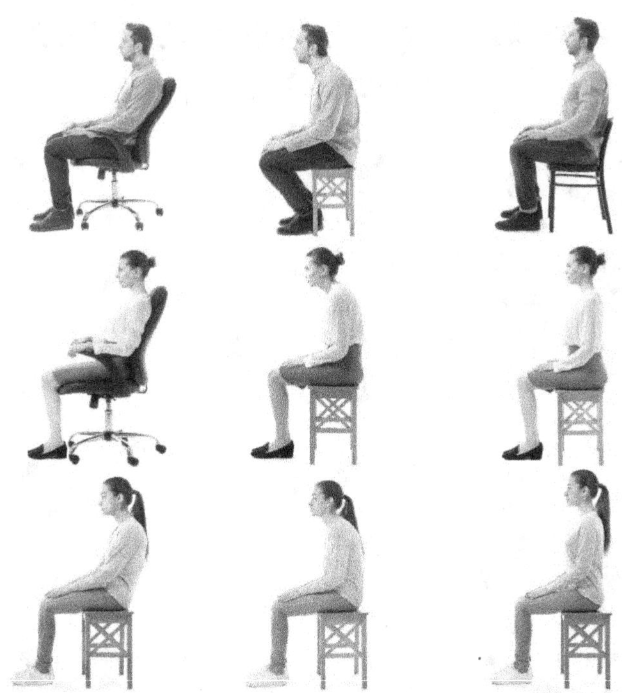

Ideal Posture When Seated

POSTURAL STRATEGIES: (A quick fix)

1. Stand with your back against the wall. The back portion of your head, shoulder blades and buttocks should touch and feel the wall, heels a few inches away from the wall.

2. Imagine a plumb from the ceiling aligned to your ear, middle of the shoulder, hip knee, and ankle. This allows less loading on the spine and joints.

3. Now, walk away from the wall, imagine carrying a book on your head. For my patients, I instruct them to visualize wearing a crown!

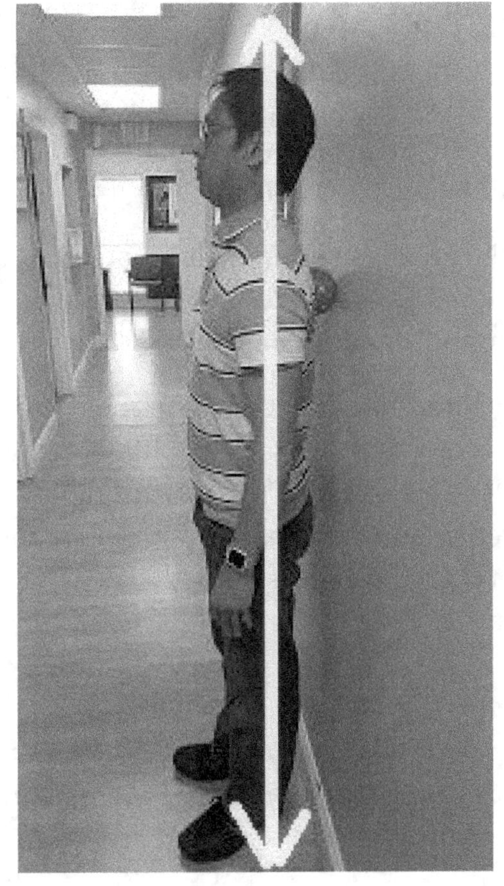

My apologies for the image quality. I just wanted to present this concept. This image is of my very shy brother-in-law whose elbow I had to twist to pose for me!

Keep shoulders relaxed and not rounded (protraction). Rounding shoulders in front does not only shorten the pectoral muscles, but also makes the muscles of the upper back and neck go into spasms. The tightening and shortening of these muscles compress the cervical spine, discs, nerve roots and limit circulation to the head. This can predispose one to headaches.

Another implication that I see prevalent in the elderly is the restriction of movement to the ribcage. Such movement is fundamental for lung expansion. Weak oxygen exchange in the body, as we know, causes fatigue, decreased alertness, decreased reflexes and protective righting reactions.

I will keep this topic concise as I have discussed this in detail in my Book 2 of the Self-Treating Patient Series.

PHYSICAL THERAPY

Physical therapists can provide valuable advice and education on various strategies to prevent or control pain symptoms stemming from muscle tension, stiff joints, and pain syndromes.

One may not be referred directly to Physical Therapy just for the headache itself. More often than not, it is associated with the primary complaints of neck pain, back pain, and shoulder pain.

Once we, as therapists, treat the musculoskeletal component of a patient's condition, the headache is alleviated and often eliminated. A physical therapist utilizes therapeutic exercises, manual therapeutic techniques, modalities for pain relief, and ongoing patient education to empower the patient to be a part of his wellness.

DISCLAIMER

Always get clearance from your physician or advice from a medical/health professional before embarking on any exercise program. Consult with your physician or get evaluated by a physical therapist to determine safe exercise parameters based on your diagnosis or condition.

SIMPLE EXERCISES TO TENSION RELIEF IN THE HEAD, NECK, AND UPPER BACK

The following exercises seem mundane and are overlooked often. If practiced daily at home or work, even for a healthy individual, the result is noticeable.

These exercises mobilize the shoulder blade, the shoulders, and the muscles of the upper back and neck. Combined with proper education and teaching on appropriate posture, patients report of almost instantaneous muscle relaxation and a lessened sense of pressure in the head.

****

SHOULDER SHRUGS

This can be done by either sitting or standing at home or the office. With the observance and awareness for good posture, these simple strategies can make a difference in one's day.

These exercises mobilize the shoulder girdle complex. Moreover, it also decrease muscle hypertonicity to allow neck motions, restore joint play, decrease tension and congestion felt in the head.

Subsequently, there is improved circulation and oxygen supply to the head and brain.

1. Keep the shoulders relaxed, place hands on both sides with the elbows extended, not bent.
2. Bring both shoulders towards the ears slowly, hold it for five (5) seconds. Bring it back down to initial position while relaxing the shoulders.
3. Repeat this exercise anywhere from 10 to 20 times, and as frequently as you can throughout the day. Especially so when you feel tight and tense on the upper back and neck.

SHOULDER CIRCLES

1. Keep the shoulders relaxed, place hands on both sides with the elbows extended, not bent.
2. Move both shoulders up, forward, down, and backward in slow circular motions. Do this for 10 - 20 times.

3. Next, reverse the movement by going back, forming big circles with both shoulders. Do this for 10 - 20 times.

You may repeat this exercise for as many times as you can until you feel the neck and upper back muscles relax. This motion mobilizes the shoulder blades, which get stuck into the rib cage when muscles supporting it are tense.

SHOULDER BLADE SQUEEZES

1. Keep the shoulders relaxed, place hands on both sides with the elbows extended, not bent.
2. Keep the head straight.
3. Lifting both shoulders towards the ears in a shrug, bring both shoulders towards the back and squeeze both shoulder blades. Hold this for 5 to 10 seconds, then relax. Repeat this exercise for about 10 - 20 times as tolerated.

It is recommended to incorporate breathing exercises during the performance of these exercises. Breathing IN through the nose and breathing OUT through the mouth. It promotes relaxation and better health.

WALL STRETCHES

Whether at home, at work, or even outside, you can easily find a wall or any standing structure to lean on. This can be your car, a bench, a tree, or just about anything. Just make sure it is fixated and does not move when you do this exercise.

1. Stand in front of a wall: place feet apart about shoulder width.
2. Place both hands on the wall in front, about waist level.

3. With both palms against the wall, slide both arms overhead. Hold this at a minimum of 5 seconds. Repeat 10 - 20 times as tolerated.

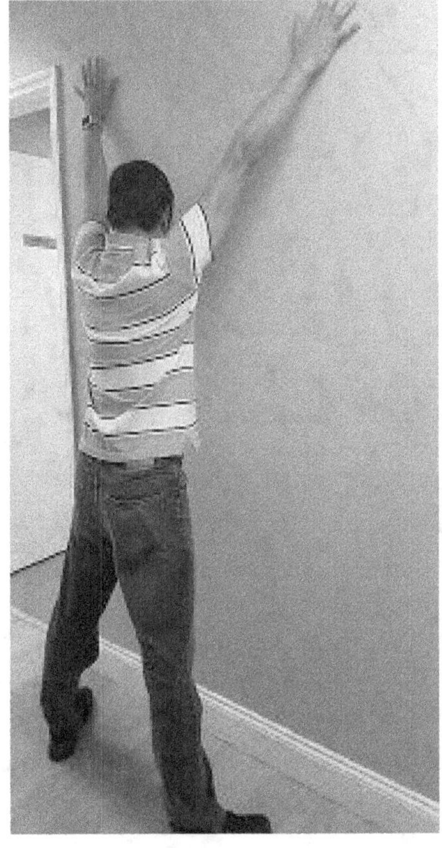

For comfort, you may also assume a "V" position of both arms above the head for shoulder joint comfort and better tolerance.

Some individuals may not have the shoulder range of motion to reach high. Just go as high as your shoulders will allow. This move can also improve the shoulder range of motion, decrease tension in the lower back, elongate the spine and promote orientation closer to midline.

Maintain position at the highest tolerated range overhead. Hold this for 5 seconds.

Repeat the exercise 10 times or more or as tolerated. Do fewer repetitions if it is too much or pain and discomfort is felt in the shoulders or neck. Mild soreness or stretch felt is okay. Anything more than the usual, one should exercise caution.

NOTE: The key is to perform this exercise within your limitations. Being a Self-Treating Patient, you know best what your body can handle.

THE NECK TOWEL ROLL TECHNIQUE

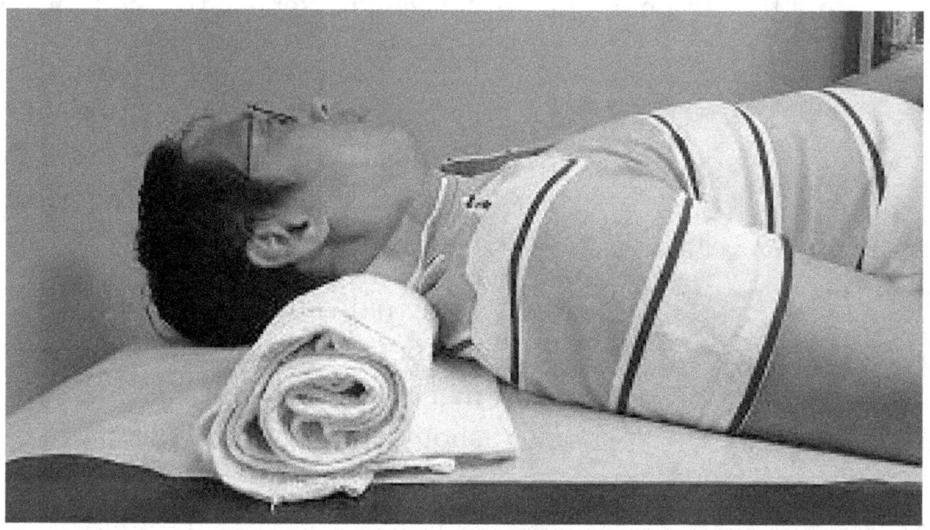

This simple at-home strategy is inexpensive and practical. The towel is adjustable. The rolled towel can be adjusted to fit your neck when lying on your back. The trick is to position the rolled towel in the curve of your neck. It should feel comfortable.

Find that sweet spot until you feel a gentle stretch, but with the feel of the neck support. Patients always ask me the ideal place to do this exercise. The floor or bed? Whatever a person's preference is and what feels comfortable. If one decides to do it on the floor, make sure getting up is not difficult.

When in the supine position, place a pillow under the knees. Keep it bent to avoid strain to the lumbar region, especially for individuals with back problems.

1. Extend your neck back (extension) over the towel roll at a comfortable range. Hold it there for at least 5 seconds.

2. As you go back to the original position, tuck your chin (neck retraction, not flexion) but do not lift the head off the roll. Hold this for 5 seconds also. Repeat this for 10 - 20 times as per your tolerance.

3. Back in a resting position over the roll, slowly turn your neck towards the right side. Hold it there for 5 seconds while allowing your neck to relax over the towel roll. Repeat this move towards the left side this time, hold this position again for 5 seconds. Repeat for 10-20 times as tolerated.

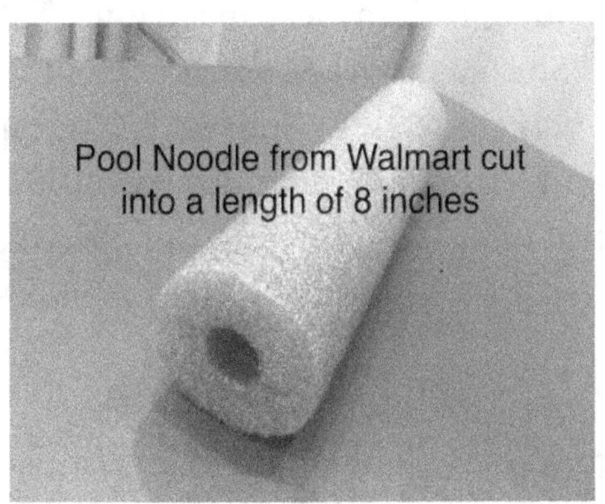

A pool noodle can also be used to support the neck while doing these exercises. Just wrap the pool noodle with a towel or any soft and comfortable piece of cloth.

****

OTHER PHYSICAL THERAPY APPROACHES

Manual Therapeutics

Many physical therapists are trained and certified in Skilled Manual Therapeutics. There are higher-level mastery and specialization in this area which takes years to accomplish.

-IASTM (Instrument Assisted Soft Tissue Mobilization), MET (Muscle Energy Techniques), MFR (Myofascial Release), Strain/Counterstrain, Nerve Manipulation, Neural Tension Release, Motion Release, Lymphatic Drainage, Trigger Point Therapy.

There are many more techniques that a physical therapist can utilize to address a specific problem. The advantage of manual treatment is that, it directly corrects the problem by skilled manipulation of soft tissue structures and joints to restore tone, motion or joint play. It is not just "massage", which is typically misconstrued.

Dina Smith, DPT, states that headaches can be caused by a lateral shift of the C1 cervical vertebra. She has worked with patients with this type of issue and corrects it using a Muscle Energy Technique or MET to restore alignment and alleviate symptoms. Different practitioners utilize specific strategies to address deficits that a patient presents with.

Dry Needling

Dry needling (also known as trigger point dry needling, intramuscular manual therapy) is now practiced by physical therapists certified in the procedure. A question always arises whether dry needling is acupuncture. Both use a filiform needle inserted into the skin to relieve pain and spasms. Dry needling practitioners use MFTPs (Myofascial Trigger Points) in the muscle while acupuncturists state they treat acupuncture points to release and enable the flow of chi.

Disregarding this debate, both are both beneficial to pain sufferers. With physical therapists, however, dry needling is just a component of the practice in treating pain and also uses modalities, manual therapeutics, to treat neuromuscular, musculoskeletal, and movement impairments.

NOTE: Dry needling is recognized as a scope of PT practice in these states: Alabama, Arizona, Colorado, the District

of Columbia, Georgia, Iowa, Kentucky, Maryland, Mississippi,

Montana, Louisiana, Massachusetts, Nevada, New Hampshire,

New Mexico, North Carolina, Ohio, *Oregon, South Carolina, Tennessee, Texas, Virginia, West Virginia, Wisconsin, and Wyoming.

Five state boards — Idaho, Kansas, Idaho, New York, and South Dakota, — have stated it is not within the scope of practice. It is not part of the scope of practice in Hawaii, as the Hawaii Physical therapy statute contains language prohibiting physical therapists from puncturing the skin for any purpose.

(Source: APTA Educational Resource Paper on PT's and Dry Needling, 2014)

Dry needling addresses migraines/headaches by dry and sterile needle insertion into the spastic, tight and painful areas in the temples and neck. In headaches, commonly affected are the temporalis, masseters, trapezius and the levator scapulae. Dry needling help ease the tension in these muscles that alleviate problems.

Physical therapists also provide education on lifestyle changes, postural correction, and task modifications at home and at the workplace to manage headache symptoms.

Modalities - Heat /Cold Packs

There is always an ongoing debate about the use of heat or cold. This is still the first question that a patient asks me.

"Do I use heat or cold?"

My personal take on the matter is that, HEAT expands: therefore it promotes local circulation and movement of the lymphatic system. COLD/ICE/COLD PACKS, on the other hand, is for vasoconstriction, meaning it results in the constriction of blood vessels.

If one has an inflamed joint that is warm to touch, swollen and effused, I recommend cold. This is also true with someone who has an acute pain from bruising, post-operative tenderness, and sensitivity. Cold Therapy is generally used in migraines as there is dilation of the arteries involved. I have had patients who are migraine sufferers who swear by the use of heat versus cold for migraines.

In the context of things, I leave it to the users to determine which of the two gives them the best relief, keeping in mind the basic properties of each.

Heating pads, hot packs, heat packs are now readily available online. I personally prefer the plug-in kind versus the microwaveable ones. I have two heat pads myself, one for the neck and a King Size piece for my back which I purchased from Amazon. It is the Sunbeam Brand. There are many brands available, just pick ones which have the automatic shut-off feature for safety and avoiding burns. It does work!

Cold packs likewise can be bought online. Let's just say I am an Amazon Prime girl. I always refer patients to purchase specific items on Amazon for years ago. If I make a commission for every patient I referred to buy supplies, I'd have a decent-sized chunk of cash!

There are gel packs however that harden once frozen. It is uncomfortable to use, and it is difficult to apply to an irregularly shaped body part such as the shoulders. Check the different products and reviews before you buy it. The Chattanooga ColPac and the FlexiKold gel ice packs remain flexible when frozen.

TIP: Wrapping the cold pack in a pillowcase is better than with a towel. A towel is too thick, and you would not get the maximum benefit of the cold pack.

Cold packs are being sold online specific for headaches, marketed as for migraines. In fact, that is suited to the contour of the head. Some patients said it has helped them tremendously.

If not available on hand a conventional cold pack, even a frozen bag of peas or corn will do just fine. Just place this around the temporal region, back of the neck and forehead. With cold pack treatment, 20 minutes seem to work just fine for most people.

Check the spot regularly with the use of heat or cold. Some individuals have impaired sensations and may get burned.

DISCLAIMER

I am not an affiliate of the companies selling the products I mention in this book, nor do I endorse these products for compensation, either monetary or in kind. These are products that my patients and I have used and is for informational purposes only. Thank you.

STYROFOAM CUP ICE MASSAGE

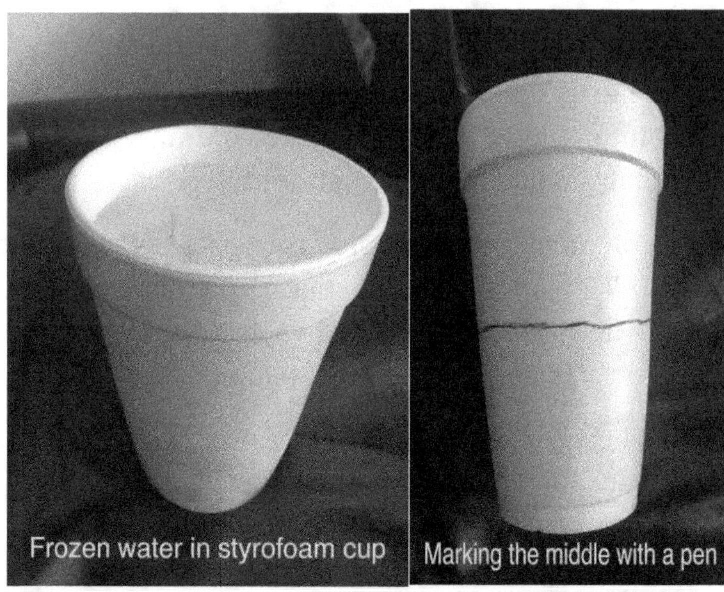

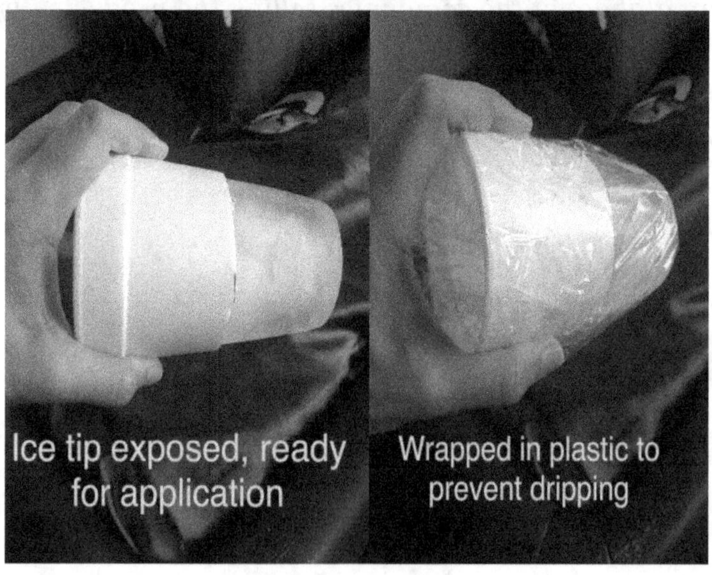

This is a practical trick to use at home for direct cryo treatment to a painful and swollen body part like the knees, ankles, elbows, or shoulders.

There are instances where an ice pack is not enough to cool off a painful joint. Direct ice massage is beneficial because it also provides a gentle pressure that improves the lymphatic flow in the area aside from the cryo effect itself. I found that circular motions in applying this to the area are more soothing and tolerable for the patient.

HERES'S HOW TO MAKE A STYROFOAM CRYO-CUP:

1. Freeze water in a styrofoam cup about 3/4th's full.

2. Once frozen, cut the styrofoam in the middle and peel off the bottom. Now you have a styrofoam handle, and the tip is the frozen ice exposed. Your hands will no longer freeze while doing the ice massage.

For headaches, you can wrap plastic around the exposed ice before doing the ice massage over painful areas such as the forehead, the temples, the back of the head (the junction between the head and neck)

Do not "freeze" the area. Over icing is not recommended. Twenty minutes at a time is a safe parameter for cold application.

Individuals with impaired sensation have to exercise caution when applying cold packs or ice packs.

THE FROZEN SPOON TRICK

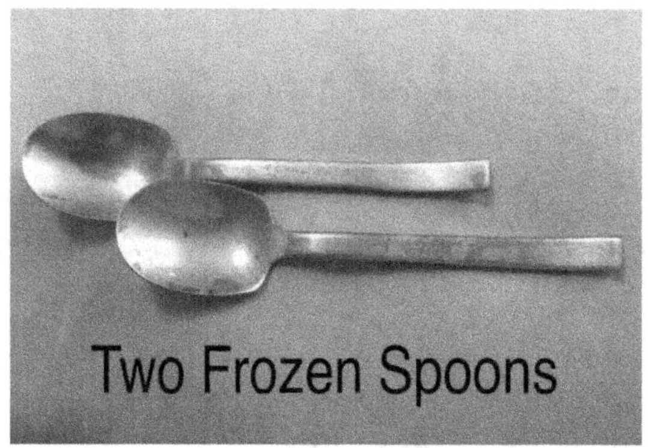

The frozen spoon trick: I learned this from one of my patients. Now, I always keep 2 frozen spoons in the freezer.

To use the frozen spoon for headaches:

Place concave side over both eyes for a few seconds, 10 - 15 seconds or as tolerated.

Place convex side to the temples next, gently pressing on the sensitive areas while gently massaging in circular motions.

Then place convex over the forehead, gently pressing in upward motions while rolling spoon over the area of the sinuses. This can really get tender and sore in this area. Just control the pressure, as per your tolerance. Once the trigger point gets deactivated from the pressure, you can tolerate this better.

Place and press convex side of the spoon at the base of the head, extending into the carotids. DO NOT PRESS TOO HARD NOR KEEP SPOONS STATIONARY IN THE CAROTIDS. You will pass out. Again, lightly press and roll in upwards, downwards and circular motions until soreness lessens.

You can freeze 4 spoons at the same time so you can exchange the used pair for a fresh one if you need more time to get relief.

****

BIOFREEZE

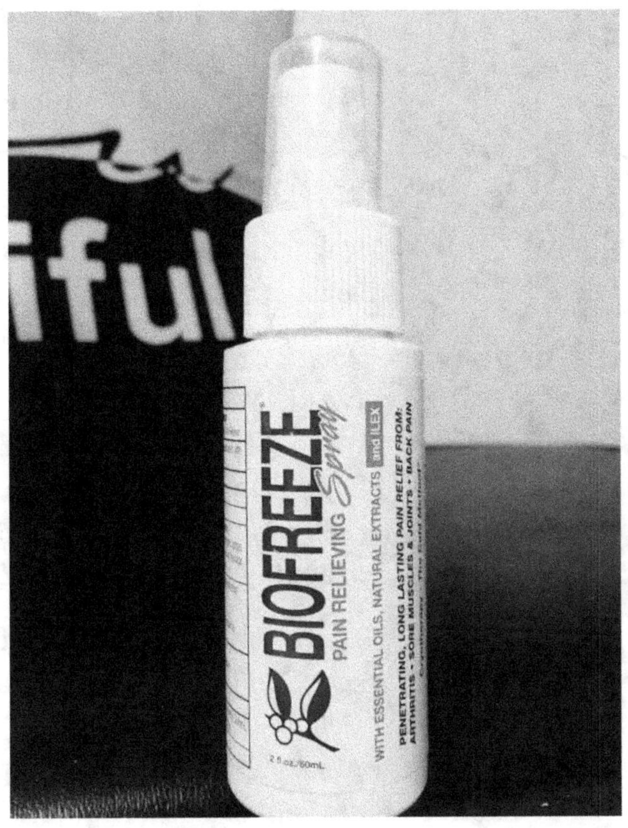

When at work or away from home, one may not readily have access to an ice pack. The Solution? BIOFREEZE.

I won't be shy. I am a big fan of Biofreeze. This small spray bottle I always carry with me, especially in my tennis bag. The cooling effect is instantaneous. It helps patients with joint replacement surgeries deal with the discomfort from swollen and warm joints. It works for everyday aches and pains.

For a headache, I have tried doing a simple trigger point therapy, (that is, applying specific cycles of pressure in the area treated) using

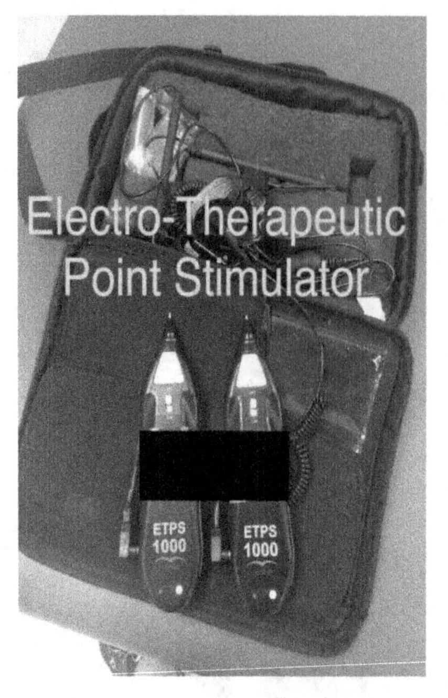

Biofreeze. I do this controlled pressure in circular motions right at the junction of the head and neck, over the very painful and tender areas. I regulate the pressure according to a person's tolerance.

It works better when the surrounding spastic and tight muscles of the neck and head are also worked on.

WARNING: Do not touch your eyes while you have this product in your hands. In fact, I use gloves as they really can feel freezing, then I start dropping things.

There is a myriad of cooling and heating pain gels on the market: Sombra, Emu, Arnicare, Bengay, Aspercreme, China Gel, Ted's Gel, Blue, Perform Gel, Arctic Relief, Mineral Ice and a lot more. On Amazon, just search for "pain gels" or "pain creams." I have noticed that there is also a proliferation of hemp cream lately. I have not personally tried these myself, but some patients and users have mentioned that it has worked for them.

Electrotherapy (ETPS)

Many Physical Therapists are certified and trained in the use of ETPS (Electrotherapeutic Point Stimulator. ETPS is a microcurrent stimulator that combines the principles of acupuncture and nerve stimulation. It is non-invasive and delivers precise stimulation to specific neuromuscular junctions and trigger areas for optimum effect. It is prescribed for the treatment of neck pain, muscle spasms, arthritis, contractures, and scar tissues, even post-surgical conditions. When the primary problem is addressed and muscles are restored to its usual tone, headache being a secondary symptom, is also relieved.

Shawky Ali, MSPT, a certified manual therapist and certified in ETPS, states that using this modality on tender points over irritated tissues has made a difference in his practice. Patients experience a 50% to 70% reduction of pain on pressure. A resulting increase in range of motion over joints involved is seen almost immediately after treatment. This is due to an increase in the muscle's firing capability.

You can ask for this specific treatment at your local Physical Therapy Outpatient clinics. You will likely find a PT who is a certified ETPS clinician.

Ultrasonic Therapy

I call therapeutic ultrasound an ancient physical rehab tool as it has been used for ages and is a go-to treatment for pain syndromes. Ultrasound, (unlike the diagnostic type used to check an unborn child in a mother's womb), is a deep heating modality. It is theorized to cause stable cavitation deep in the tissues that speed up the healing process.

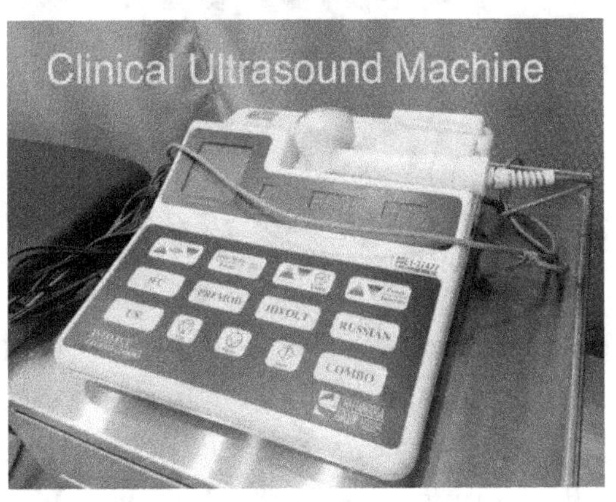

Available portable units are being sold in the market anywhere from $89 to $250. Again, I do keep one myself on hand for personal use if I need it. Now, still, because you hardly feel anything during the application, it is hard to determine how well it works. I use it on very tight shoulder muscles, calves, ankles, the bottom of the foot (for plantar fasciitis) or the back. If you do purchase one for home use, follow the instructions and precautions well.

Once I do use it on very tight muscles, especially of the neck and shoulders, it does relieve a headache in conjunction with other alternative treatments.

TRANSCUTANEOUS ELECTRICAL NERVE STIMULATOR (TENS)

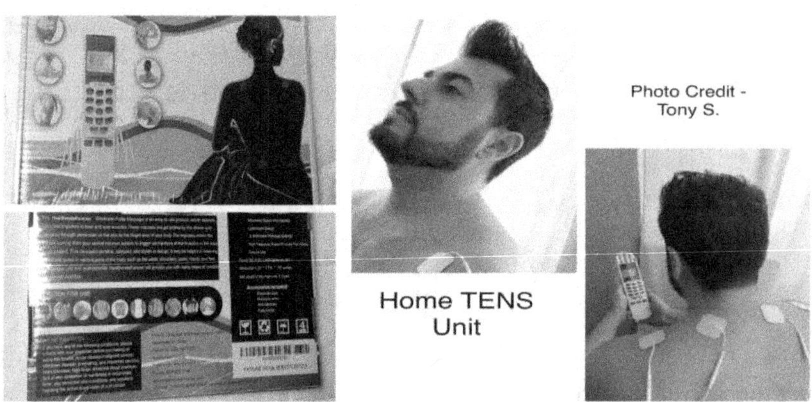

(Above image shows my preferred placement of 4 pads at the back for headache relief)

Many years ago, TENS units were mostly available from medical supplies companies as it was easily reimbursed by insurance payers. They were costly. It also required a doctor's prescription and explanation of the medical necessity for it to be covered.

Recently, insurance coverage and the process of getting TENS units covered has become complicated.

The hoops that one has to go through for a TENS unit to be covered by insurance is no longer worth the hassle.

It is surprising that a large percentage of my patients are not aware of the home unit TENS / Electrical Stimulators now readily available in the market.

Again, Amazon carries a lot of these units with different features and models. They are convenient and portable. Most units can be hooked up to a belt loop or placed in a pocket.

They vary in sizes, the smallest I have seen so far is the size of a credit card and is very light. Many are USB rechargeable, some use regular AA or AAA batteries. There are more sophisticated units that are wireless.

I am handicapped when it comes to technology, and my brain prefers the user-friendly, easy to operate ones. One of my patients brought in a wireless model she bought at a health and wellness expo. She adds that it cost her about $300. To this day, we still couldn't make it work between the three of us, including her boyfriend.

So she bought one online for $25, and it worked great for her.

Just search for "TENS units" on Amazon, Google or any online store, and you will be amazed at the number of models and units that are available nowadays.

Most of these units are FDA approved as they are marketed as "massagers" at times. There are more complex brands. Just pick one that is simple, easy to operate, and is compact. Read the reviews. It's amazing how you learn a lot from the reviews.

When using these tiny gadgets, however, heed the precautions, proper and safe use. **Read and follow the instructions carefully.**

TENS units alleviate pain by delivering electrical impulses to the skin, thereby flooding the nervous system. This decreases the transmission of pain signals to the spinal cord, and the brain also called the pain gate theory.

Another benefit is the promotion of local circulation that is theorized to help release endorphins, the body's natural pain killers.

The image is an actual image of a unit I use personally. I must have bought dozens of this unit and gave it away to friends as a present. I have also brought many during my medical mission and donated it to select groups who participated and volunteered.

I have referred many patients to get this on Amazon for the last 5 years. As of 10/02/2019, the prize has gone up to $29.99. It used to be only $23.49. It is still worth the price for all the features you get.

I reiterate I am not endorsing any product for favors. I just happened to have used this model, and it has always served my patients and me well. It doesn't matter which model you use, they have one thing in common: they do work for pain relief by decreasing muscle spasm, promoting local circulation and inducing muscle relaxation which is beneficial for headaches.

Do read the contraindications and instructions well before usage. Observe all precautions.

ACUPOINT PENS

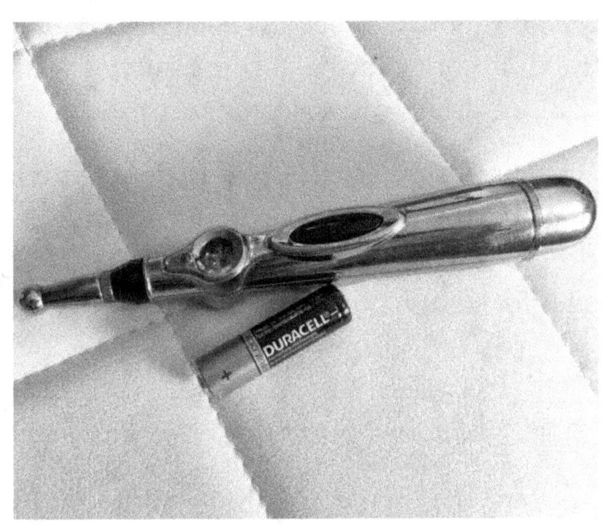

Widely known as electronic Acupuncture Pen, Energy Release Pen, Meridian Pen. I prefer to call it ACU-pens, as ACU-puncture doesn't sound right. There is really no "puncturing" that is happening with this pen.

It is non-invasive and does not penetrate the skin. It is merely a point that comes in contact with the skin, and where electrical impulses are conducted to the skin over trigger points.

This tiny contraption was impressive. For its size, it can generate significant contractions in the muscles stimulated. One was brought in by a patient who swears by this for her headaches and muscle pains.

Curious, I did order one to try. I remember paying about $17 for the model and type I got pictured here. It was easy to operate although instructions were pretty bad. I had to research other models online just to get some sound instructions on how to use it.

I admit I hated the way it felt at first as the electrical impulse delivered was strong! It felt like I being electrocuted with tiny shocks that made the muscles contract strongly even to the point of pulling my head some to the side repeatedly.

However, the result was unexpected. It relieved my headache! I directed the point to the trigger areas at the base of my neck and the tight upper trapezius muscles for about 30 seconds each area. You do feel the strong muscle contractions jerk your head some. After a while, however, that weird electrical sensation was welcome torture!

This is my personal experience and some friends and patients. It may not be for everybody. It may be too intense for some people. But again, I share this information for the reader to decide whether to try it or not and just to provided information on what's out there.

Kinesiotaping

(Photo Credit to Mr. Tim Standifer)

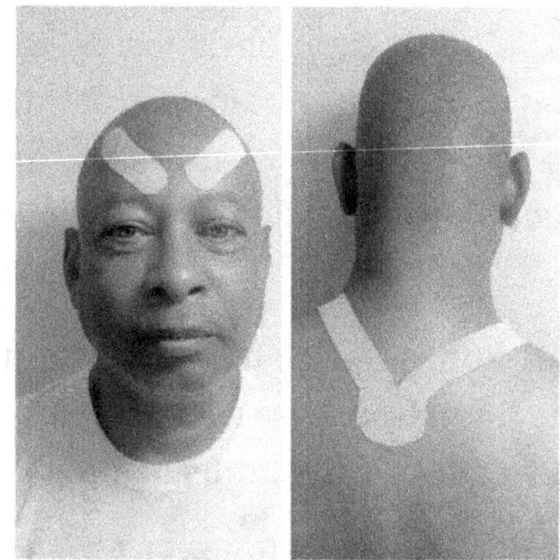

The onset of Kinesiotaping has provided a whole new dimension to the physical rehabilitation world. Dr. Kenzo Kaze, Jim Walls and Tsuyoshi Takashi as illustrated in the second edition of their clinical reference book for Kinesiotaping, featured a taping for muscle -contraction headache that can happen when the head and neck is flexed forward from a deviant posture and stresses of everyday life and at work.

Both taping methods above enables a decrease in muscle tension, in conjunction with postural correction. On the right is a simple taping technique to decrease tension in the muscles of the neck. The ideal placement of the tape behind the neck is higher and over the splenius capitis muscles, but this patient prefers this placement.

There are many other brands of Kinesio Tapes that have come up. The most convenient to use is the pre-cut type which makes it easier for an untrained person to apply. There are specific techniques for application, however, and physical therapists and other physical rehabilitation professionals receive specialized training and certification for the method to be correct and valid. It requires an extensive understanding of human anatomy and biomechanics.

You may look up online resources on how to apply the KT tape if you decide to do it on your own. Or better yet, ask a clinical person trained in a proper application, so you can carry it out by yourself at home.

For my patients who are more active or athletic, I do show them basic application techniques for their specific issues. Once taught, they were able to apply it decently and have reported of having relief.

One advantage of the KT tape is that it can stay on the skin for 3-4 days. Before the application of the KT tape, however, remember to clean the area of the body's natural oils or lotion or the tape will not stick. An alcohol pad will do the trick. One can still take a shower with it on, just do not rub soap or shower gel over it. After showering, just tap the taped area with a dry towel. Do not rub it up and down.

ACUPUNCTURE

I will not elaborate so much on acupuncture. It is a popular Chines medicinal art. It is now widely accepted in the medical world. Thin needles are inserted into specific parts of the body said to restore the flow of Qi, stimulate relaxation, and promote healing.

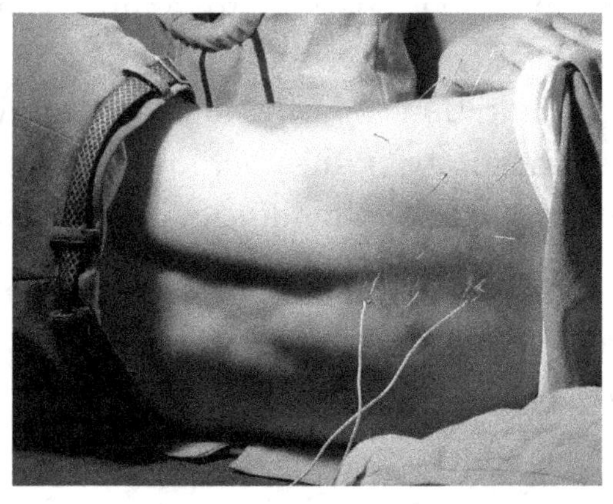

Many of my patients have indeed received acupuncture treatment. More than 60 percent stated it worked for them. Some have reported significant relief from headaches.

MASSAGE THERAPY

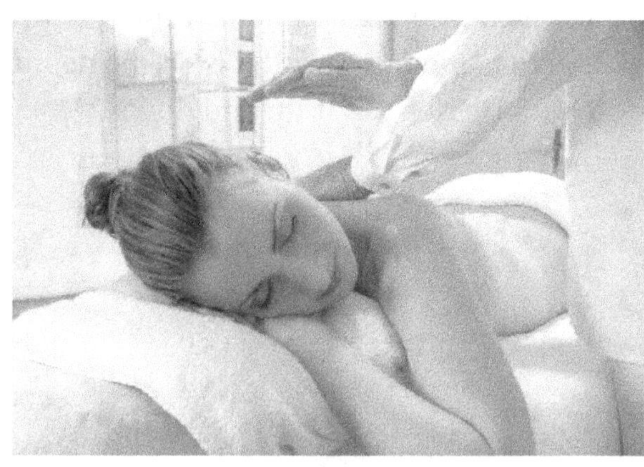

Ahhhh, the exhilarating feeling you get after a good massage. It is a fact that it brings ultimate relaxation, decreases tension, and improves mood, among other benefits.

When the body is relaxed, stress is eliminated, and the body can function better that can aid in managing headaches.

CHIROPRACTIC CARE

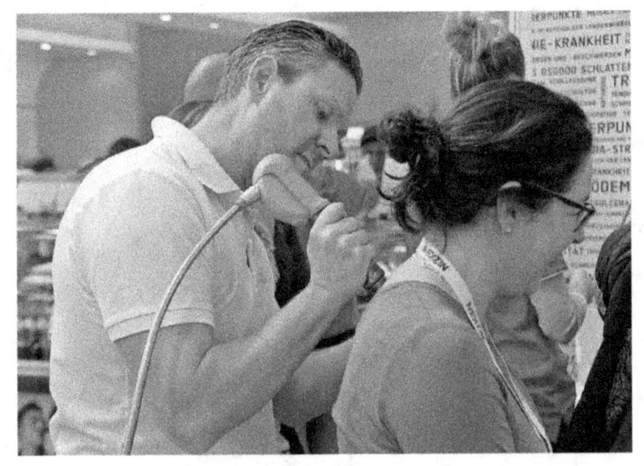

Spinal manipulation, especially on the neck, is a common approach in Chiropractic care. A few studies did indicate that this approach did benefit patients who suffer from migraine and cervicogenic headaches. Chiropractors also provide education and advice on nutrition and recommendations of vitamins.

Chiropractors nowadays are as commonplace as pharmacies. If inclined to try this type of treatment, inquire from a friend who has been to one, or read reviews.

Otherwise, you can always pick one and have a discussion with the chiropractor about your issues. People tend to go to the ones that they are most comfortable with.

HYPNOSIS

Hypnosis has been considered a valuable adjunct to certain types of physical and mental illnesses. It is also relevant in decreasing anxiety and coping with stress before a medical procedure, changing undesirable behaviors (to mention a few:

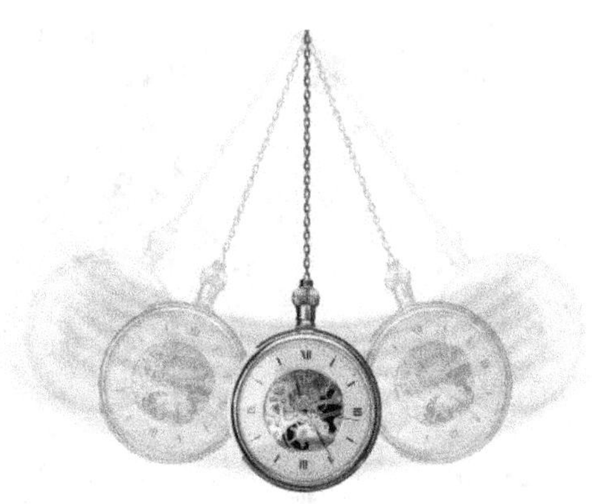

bedwetting, smoking, compulsive disorders, alcoholism, phobias, etc.), promoting desirable and healthy habits. Self-hypnosis was also mentioned under this category.

In a Mayo Clinic Health newsletter, it was mentioned that when under hypnosis, a person has an elevated state of concentration and focus while in a half-conscious state. One also feels very relaxed, calm, and open to suggestions. It was also stated that not everyone is susceptible to hypnosis. The more receptive a person is to hypnotherapy, the more likely one will benefit from it.

Experts say, however, that one should exercise caution when choosing hypnosis, or hypnotherapy as an alternative treatment as it does have side effects. This is not limited to dizziness, the creation of false memories, anxiety, and even depression. Consult a professional before considering this option.

ESSENTIAL OILS AND AROMATHERAPY

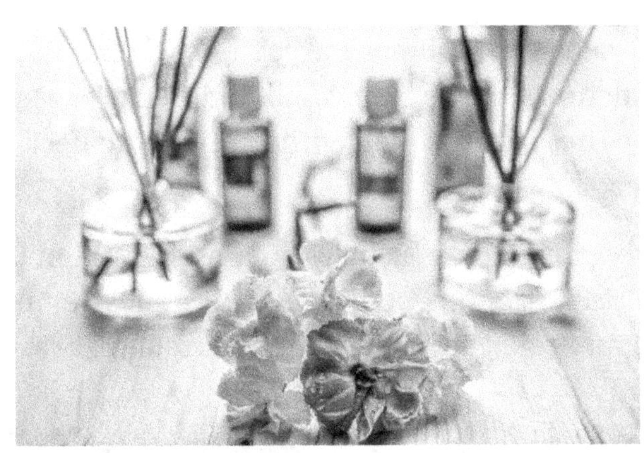

The use of essential oils was said to date back from ancient Egypt and was used for cosmetic and medicinal purposes, and even used for the embalming process.

Aromatherapy has gained roots as a holistic alternative to common ailments.

For headaches, the most popular ones are the following: Peppermint due to its menthol properties known for muscle relaxation and pain relief and is the base for most migraine headache relief sticks and roll-ons now in the market. Many are available in health stores, pharmacies, and online.

It can be inhaled via steam inhalation, directly inhaling its vapors, applied directly to the skin or some sellers even recommend adding a few drops to a drink. I personally do not advocate ingesting essentials just for the reason that the risks outweigh the benefits. There are no in-depth studies that recommend the ingestion of essential oils.

I personally keep one on hand, and I daresay, for my severe attacks to the point of nausea. I have tried using a peppermint roll-on. It does the trick, combined with a simple

TRIGGER POINT self-treatment. Trigger points are areas in the body that hurt and very tender to pressure.

In headaches, one will find sensitive and sore areas in the temples, behind the ears, and the junction between the skull and neck. These can be very painful to touch. These are also felt at the base of the neck, and even at the top of the head.

The trick is to press these sensitive areas (usually holding it for about 20-30 times, then releasing pressure; repeat as needed until less pain is felt)in a cycle of pressing and releasing causing the muscle to relax and thus providing relief.

These trigger regions, however, can be very painful and sensitive to touch at first. This is to be expected. It is necessary to start out with a tolerable amount of pressure or circular motions in the area until one's tolerance builds up. With continuous and rhythmic cycles of pressure in the area, the trigger point gets deactivated and becomes less sensitive to applied pressure and touch.

There is a horde of information and articles available about trigger point readily available.

Other essential oils known to help with headaches are Lavender Oil, Chamomile, Eucalyptus, Rosemary, Sage, Geranium, Citrus, Frankincense. There is little study, however, on which essential oil is suited to each specific headache type.

My patients shared their personal experiences with the use of essential oil for headaches. All of them have used different types but did a report of relief with their specific choice.

MEDITATION

Meditation is a known practice by Buddhist monks to cultivate inner balance, promoting calmness, well-being, mental clarity, and emotionally stable state.

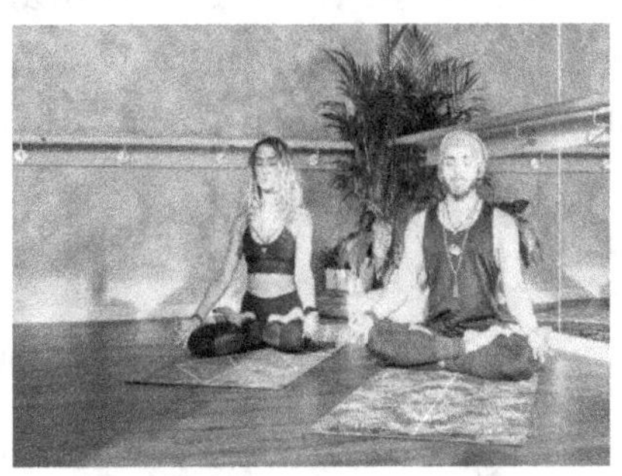

Depending on the type of meditation practiced, target results are achieved. In general, it promotes relaxation, decreased anxiety, improved concentration, and inner harmony.

Chi Gong and Tai Chi are considered a "walking or moving meditation." There are many types of meditation: Mindfulness Meditation, Concentration Meditation, Transcendental, Zen meditation, Kundalini Yoga, Breath Awareness Meditation, Progressive Relaxation Meditation. There are many more types of meditation practiced by individuals. The aforementioned is the most common. No matter what type one practices for the intended result, benefits are significant.

Short term benefits of meditation include but are not limited to: longer-lasting relaxation, decreased anxiety, improved alertness, and concentration, reduced heart rate, calmer breathing, and improved one's sense of well - being.

SIMPLE GUIDE TO MEDITATION:

1. Find a quiet place to meditate. You can either lie down or sit, eyes closed. I find that I do better with meditation or ZEN music of choice. YouTube alone has myriads of this type of music.

2. Focus and "feel" the movement of your body when you inhale or exhale. The motion of the shoulders, ribcage, and abdomen is expanding, moving. Breathe naturally, calmly.

For a beginner, two to three minutes is sufficient. As you get better at concentration, you will find that the time you stay in meditation increases.

One can always research for advanced meditation techniques if further pursuit of this practice is desired.

FLOTATION THERAPY

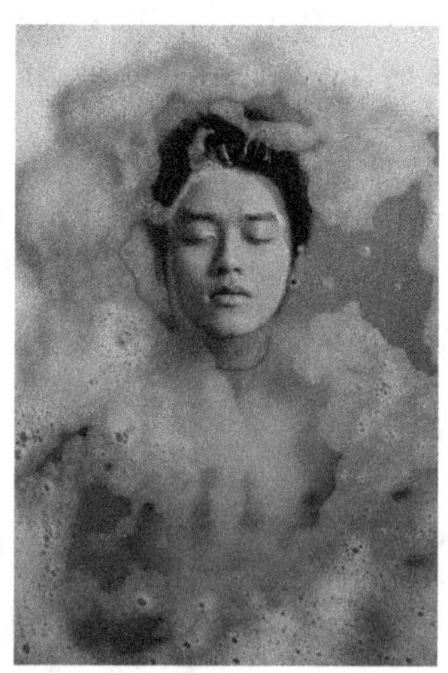

Flotation therapy, also known as floating, is a trending relaxation practice where a flotation tank, a float pod, or a sensory deprivation chamber is used. A controlled study revealed that subjects who used flotation as relaxation showed a significant decrease in blood pressure, both systolic and diastolic, versus the group of subjects who practiced the same relaxation technique in the same position without flotation. It is now prevalent in spas and wellness centers.

The flotation pod is filled with water at body temperature and suffused with about a thousand pounds of Epsom salts. This allows the body to float due to its density. The time in the pod usually lasts from 60 - 90 minutes.

Most people report a deep relaxation, a heightened "letting go feeling" that is very calming. There are a few however who are claustrophobic and swore they'd never do it again. Flotation therapy is now mainstream, and one can always check with local wellness centers and spas if they offer this at their facility.

CRYOTHERAPY

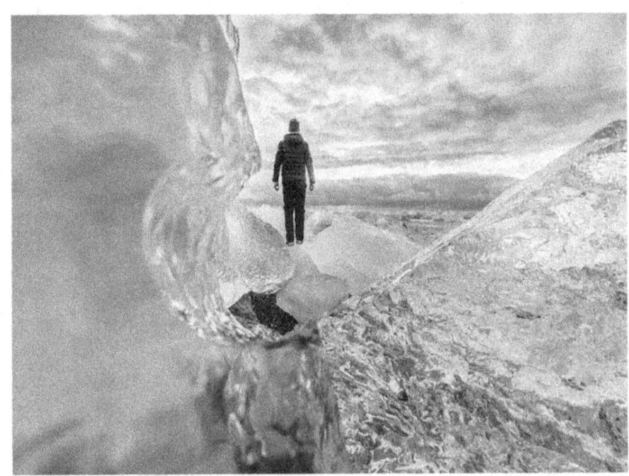

Cryotherapy in this topic pertains to whole body submersion in an ice tank or chamber that is minus 200 degrees or more for a few minutes (2 - 4 minutes). Local chiropractic, massage clinics, gyms, and wellness centers now offer this non-medical treatment.

Although there are not a lot of studies done for its benefits, its known benefits indicate that it helps with pain relief and muscle healing. This is especially so with athletic injuries. There no official studies were done on its effect on headaches. Cold treatment or cryo treatment directed to the head and neck did ease symptoms of migraine headaches but did not prevent it.

Although controversial, mentioned benefits of cryotherapy included pain relief from arthritis, reduction of migraine headache symptoms, improves mood, treats dermatitis and other skin conditions, aids with dementia, decreases the sensation of paresthesias, and may even help with low-risk tumors.

A self-study should be done before trying out this alternative treatment as there are known side effects of skin irritation, tingling or numbness.

Individuals with impaired sensation should exercise caution when trying heat or cold applications.

YOGA

Yoga originated from ancient India consisting of mental, physical, and spiritual practices. In the western world, however, it is a popular physical exercise that is posture based for relaxation and anxiety relief. The benefits of yoga practice are well known: flexibility, strength, decreased 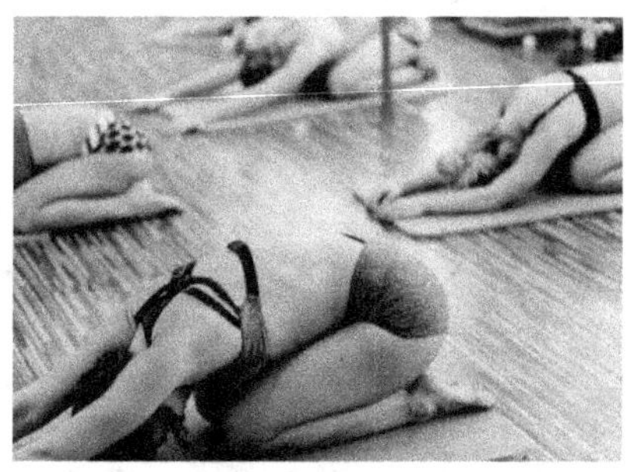 anxiety, increased energy, vitality, alertness, focus, cardiorespiratory health, weight control.

HYDROMASSAGE THERAPY

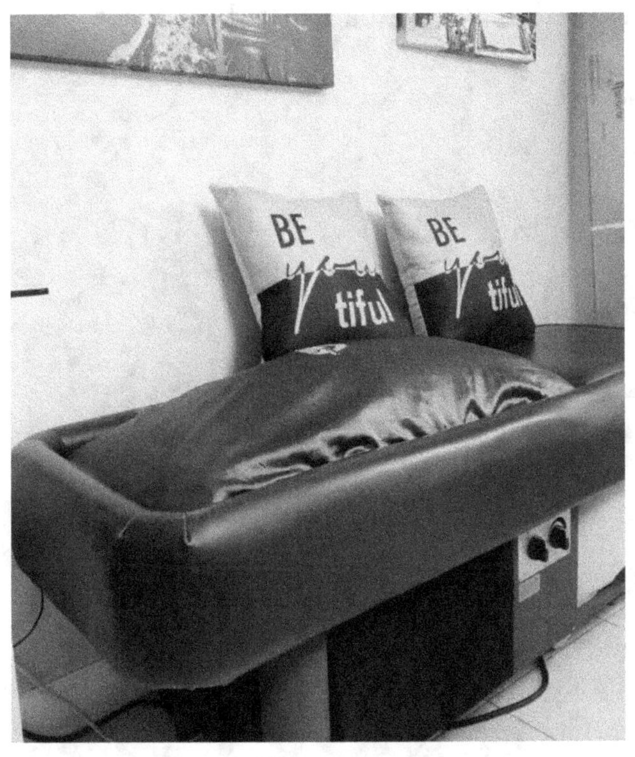

I just have to mention this as I have this unit at home. I can attest to the relief from headache pains I get once in a while. It is one of the few luxuries I indulge in.

The warm water inside the hydrobed's belly is agitated by jets inside with adjustable speed. It features a timer and adjustment for intensity. It is much needed after a hectic day at work or after an intensive game with tennis buddies.

This unit is from Sidmar, and although an older model, has served me through the years. There are newer models and different functions. Prices and features vary, and the more features you want, the pricier it gets.

The cost of hydromassage beds can range from a few thousand to twenty grand (20K) and above. I have seen used units on eBay that are below $1,000.00.

The combination of heat and agitation does wonders for muscle relaxation and promoting circulation, which in turn, can, and may also aid in general relaxation that can ease the pain from headaches.

REFLEXOLOGY

Reflexology is an ancient manual bodywork practice that involves pressing on specific points in the body corresponding to a particular organ or body part to treat certain illnesses.

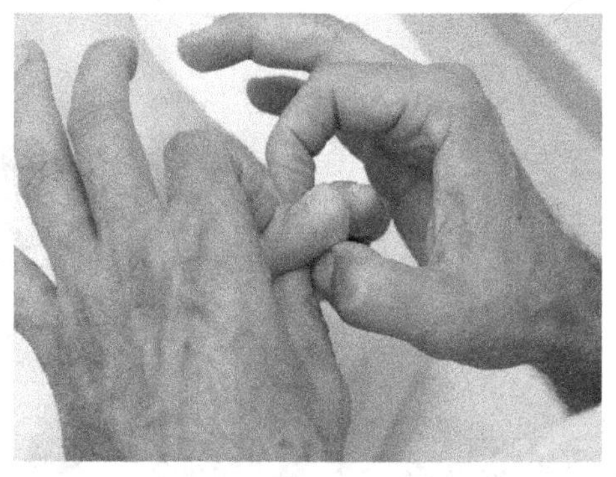

A known acupressure point for headaches is between the thumb and the index finger: that fleshy part. This area is pressed anywhere from 30 - 60 seconds and repeat as needed. Interestingly enough, a reflexology gadget clipped to this acupressure point is now sold on the market. Users and reviewers indicated that it does help relieve headaches.

Other known reflexology points include a point between the eyebrows, the temples, the inner corners of the eyes, on top of the big toes, inside the big toes.

Reflexology is now a widely accepted treatment alternative and the practice is thriving.

It is an option that may benefit some people and worth exploring, especially for chronic headache sufferers.

****

Conclusion

I n retrospect, there are always adaptations to life changes brought about by infirmities and impairments. A sufferer, a patient is left to make decisions and seek alternative treatment if traditional approaches have not brought on relief.

One must go through proper consultations and diagnostics to determine diagnoses and their implications.

If not content with the initial consult and its results, it is the patient's prerogative to seek a second opinion.

Once underlying issues are determined and proper medical treatment plan has been established, I advocate going through with the recommended method of care.

If and when a person feels that exploration of further options is necessary to alleviate symptoms that hinder daily task performance, then discussion with the treating professional is worthwhile.

One may be surprised how receptive some medical professionals are, regarding alternatives and even suggest further options.

The reason for all this is the **QUALITY OF LIFE.** When a seemingly minor pain as a headache diminishes the joy of doing the simplest tasks of daily living, then finding solutions is a must.

This is where one exercises the option of being the **SELF-TREATING PATIENT.**

Even if only one individual is enlightened by just a single useful information from this book, its purpose has been served.

From the Author

Thank you for spending time with me by reading this book!

I have had the privilege of working with patients who have surmounted physical obstacles through hard work and determination.

The resilience, determination, and motivation of these exemplary beings have inspired me to share coping strategies and ideas for augmenting Quality of Life.

Some practical ideas shared in this book are from this group of individuals. The simplicity of utilizing resources that are readily available at home has been helpful to others as well.

-Lovena

FUTURE RELEASES IN THE SELF-TREATING PATIENT SERIES:

Book 1 - A Practical Guide to Managing Headache

Book 2 - A Practical Guide to Managing Pain by Improving Posture

Book 3 - A Practical Guide to Preventing Falls in the Elderly

Book 4 - A Practical Guide to Managing Menopause

Book 5 - A Practical Guide to Managing Fibromyalgia

Book 6 - A Practical Guide to Managing Parkinson's Disease

Book 7 - A Practical Guide to Managing Falls with Tai Chi

Book 8 - A Practical Guide to Managing Stress

Book 9 - The CBD Revolution: Yay or Nay?

Book 10 - Medical Marijuana: The Hype & Controversy

Book 11 - Prime Motionz - Tai Chi based Exercises for Balance

And Fall Prevention - developed by **Lovena Suson, P.T.**

Would you like to be notified of new releases by this Author?

Get Notified Here: https://forms.gle/kLUNQRtYsm5emZjP7

To receive notifications for Free & Helpful E-books & Articles from this Author:

Get Notified Here: https://forms.gle/PzPqME3MXnKspxVi6

You can write the Author at mailto:primemotionz@gmail.com

9 781699 303061